BACK FROM BURNOUT

Seven Steps to Healing from Compassion Fatigue and Rediscovering (Y)our Heart of Care

Written by: Dr. Frank Gabrin

Clear2care's mission is to heal the everyday heroes of healthcare from the disease of compassion fatigue and burnout. We believe that caring for others should feel incredibly good and seek to dismantle the big lie, or the myth, that caregivers have been taught and incorporated into their practice that we believe is the cause of this dis-ease: The myth of keeping our professional distance in order to be better caregivers. In its place, we seek to teach that to do better we do not need to step back, but rather we need to take a step forward and connect more fully with the hurting human in front of us. When we take this step forward, we engage the protocol of True Care, which is what will cause us on both sides of the stethoscope to feel better. Learn more at: clear2care.com

In Gratitude

This is for all the souls who have ever actively cared for me. Especially when I found it difficult to care for myself when I was being treated for cancer, when I was struggling in general, or when I was so badly burned out. This is for those souls, of which there were so many, who came to point me, show me, and teach me how to find my way back to a healthy, rich, and full experience of life.

Although no list could ever be complete, I would like to thank my parents, my brother, his wife Dianne and my nephews Michael, Matt and Ryan. Without Mary, Vince, David, Shalom, Abraham, Allison, Julie, Bill, Cheryl, Bob, Debra, Ruth, Eitan, Yehuda, Michal, Michael, Monica, Karen and the Rav Berg, I probably would not be here to tell my story.

More than anything else, this work is a labor of love that I have done for you.... especially those of you who are broken by empathetic overload, fatigue and burnout. My hope is that you will use these steps that I have learned to bring you back home to the individual you've always wanted to be, for herein lies your destiny.

CONTENTS

Warning: The Surgeon General Has Determined That Caring for Others Is Hazardous to Your Health

What if the application to medical or nursing school, or the packet for EMT or Paramedic training, had carried a warning like this on the first page? We probably would have ignored it. How could caring for others be bad for you? It just seems intuitively wrong. Most of us were young, idealistic and invincible when we enrolled in school. We would all have said, "Naah . . . that could never happen to me!"

But if you work in healthcare today, you probably know all too well that it *can* happen to you—and perhaps it's happening to you right now.

Whether you are in the hospital, an office, an extended-care facility, or a patient's home, you've worked hard to get where you are. You've invested so much of yourself in becoming a nurse, a physician, a hospitalist, a manager, a medic or an aide; you studied, you trained, then you trained some more; you invested yourself and your life fully into your job. And some days it is so great you want to pinch yourself.

You and I both know there is nothing more satisfying than helping someone, especially when the outcome is good and the help is appreciated. There really is nothing better, except—well, maybe—

chocolate or great sex. But those glimpses of greatness have diminished over time, and now they seem to come further and further apart. Those passing moments of satisfaction just aren't enough, and most of the time you are not feeling so good.

Our healthcare workdays can be brutal, whatever clinical setting we work in. Patients can be entitled, ungrateful and sometimes just downright rude. Co-workers can be inflexible, uncooperative and sometimes ruder than the patients. What is expected of us is, well, unbelievable. My bet is that you feel you're working harder than ever, but at the end of the day, you are more drained, exhausted and frustrated than ever, with nothing left to give to yourself or your family. To put it bluntly, you're burned out. You may be afraid to say it out loud, but some part of you is wondering, *Is this as good as it gets?*

Malcolm Gladwell tells us in his famous and well-respected book *Outliers* that in order to achieve mastery at anything, one needs to practice it for at least 10,000 hours. Well, let's take emergency physicians. Once they are finished with their training, they work roughly three twelve-hour shifts a week, on average. So for the average emergency physician to become a master of his or her craft, he or she would need to work 833 twelve-hour shifts, and at three shifts a week, that would take 277 weeks. Which would mean that to be masters of emergency medicine, all these young men and women would have to do is work consistently in the emergency department as the attending physician for five and a half years. At that point, they should most definitely be at the top of their game, and you'd think that would feel pretty good about all they have accomplished and all the good they do.

Instead, studies show us, two out of three of our Emergency Physicians are experiencing at least one symptom of burnout. Something similar is happening in other medical specialties—general internists, family practice physicians and neurologists rank 2, 3, and 4 on the most-burned-out-physicians list. This same situation is also affecting our bright and dedicated mid-level providers, nurses, techs, medics, firemen and social workers.

When I went to the literature, I was surprised to find that this is not a uniquely American phenomenon. The same thing is happening in Germany, Canada, Iran and even as far away as Australia. It seems that this phenomenon is universal among those who choose to help others: something overrides the feeling of mastery, the feeling you *deserve* to have that you're at the top of your game. That "something" happens in no other segment of the industrial workforce. That "something" only happens to care givers. We've given that something the name "compassion fatigue," and we know that if compassion fatigue is left untreated, it inevitably grows into professional burnout. And it may surprise you to learn that both of these maladies are characterized as forms of post-traumatic stress disorder, or PTSD. Think about that for a moment: it means that our choice to enter the helping professions leads us to feel and behave like victims of abuse and trauma. Does that sound right to you?

They tell us there is no cure for burnout except to take a step back—to take time off and take better care of ourselves. But **the worst thing about workplace PTSD is that its symptoms** don't just surface when you are practicing professionally, they **spill over into every aspect of your life**.

And what do these symptoms look like? If there were a warning label on that med-school application, we'd naturally expect it to spell out the dangers. Well, the literature would tell us that the price we must pay for caring for others is that one or more (perhaps even all) of the following will occur:

- We will feel deep physical and emotional exhaustion

- We will see a profound decrease in our ability to feel empathy for our patients, our co-workers and even our loved ones

- We will be irritable and quick to anger

- Our worldview will be disrupted

- We will become either hypersensitive or insensitive to emotional material, both at work and at home

- We will lose the ability to maintain close personal friendships

- We will develop problems with both emotional and physical intimacy in all of our personal relationships

- We will be more likely to divorce

- We will become cynical, especially at work

- We will come to dread working with certain types of patients, or certain patients in particular

- We will lose the ability to enjoy our jobs

- We will lose our ability to make decisions and our care for patients: we will be impaired

- We will lose interest in life itself

- We will lose our concern or respect for other people

- Our perceptions of people will become dehumanized

- We will begin to label people or groups of people in a derogatory manner

- We will have trouble sleeping

- We will develop low self esteem

- We will become clinically depressed

- We will gain or lose weight

- We will feel hopeless

- We will become more susceptible to physical illness

- We will become more likely to turn to addictions like drugs, alcohol or gambling for temporary relief

- We will be more likely than the general population to kill ourselves

I can honestly say that I have, at one point or another in my career, experienced all of these symptoms except feeling suicidal. What about you? Which symptoms have you succumbed to? If you recognized yourself in any of these lines, then this book you are reading is written just for you. Please get yourself into your favorite chair and read on, because I have something very special to share with you.

Opportunity Knocking

What are my qualifications to educate you about the hazards of making your living in the field of healthcare today? My specialty training is in the field of Emergency Medicine. I am the doctor who works the night shift, the weekends, and all the holidays at your local hospital emergency room or emergency department. I was taught to think in "worst-case scenarios", while at the same time to make a diagnosis and develop a plan of treatment for the less emergent cases. If you, as a patient, have a real medical emergency, then I am one of those well-trained, seasoned, board-certified Emergency Medicine Specialists you hope to find on duty when you roll up to the ED.

The reality is that most of my patients do not have true medical emergencies, so I see all sorts of clinical problems, as well as people who are just overwhelmed by life's problems. I don't hold any fancy titles and I am not the director of anything. But I can say that I have spent the last quarter of a century at the bedside of America's sick, injured, intoxicated, impaired and disenfranchised. The whole focus of my career has been on the people I care for, their families and the people I work with. And today I am more passionate about care, and about what I do and who I am as an emergency physician, than I have ever been.

Don't get me wrong—when I was a bright-eyed, bushy-tailed, wet-behind-the-ears young doctor, so excited about flying in on the helicopter and landing at the scene of a bad car accident and performing heroic interventions like intubating patients right there on the highway, I experienced immense passion for my work. These days, I experience that same passion for what I do in a different way. Today, I experience that passion even in the most frustrating situations, even with patients who do not have "real" emergencies, and even—*especially*—in those cases where it seems as if there is nothing I can do, nothing I have to offer except my caring.

And today, what I am most passionate about of all is caring for you, the healthcare worker at the patient's bedside: the doctor, the nurse, the medic, the social worker, the aide, the housekeeper, the registration worker, the secretary or the health unit coordinator. I know how difficult your days can be. I know how much you are hurting. I know firsthand, and I am living proof that it does not have to be that way.

You see; I was you. I *am* you. I had all sorts of problems and all sorts of excuses, reasons why I was unhappy at work. Too many patients, not enough staff, lazy staff, demanding bosses, managers who didn't even understand my problems, uncooperative specialists, demanding patients, entitlement issues, unrealistic expectations and lousy satisfaction scores. You name it, I complained about it, to myself and to just about anyone who would listen.

For a long time, I could put up with the negatives because it was so great when something positive happened. But over time the positive experiences eroded until they were few and far between, while the negative stuff seemed to happen almost always. All of that negativity can leave you feeling overburdened, unappreciated and overwhelmed, and it only stands to reason that if this is your daily experience of working in the hospital, you might just start to hate the hospital.

I used to feel this way. I literally hated going to work. I dreaded putting on my plastic, emotionless, politically correct clinical face, my scrubs, my lab coat and my stethoscope, and driving to the hospital. No matter how hard I tried to feel better, it never got any better. I felt as if I was working in a dungeon and there were dragons out to get me everywhere I turned. My situation was bleak, as yours may be. Then I discovered the utterly simple, yet thoroughly life-changing solution I'm going to share with you here.

What will you get from reading this book? Well, think about a really positive experience you had at work, perhaps when you first started your career, where you helped someone, and this person knew you had helped and thanked you for helping. How was that? How did that make you feel? What I am going to teach you is how to feel that way more and more often. You are really going to love the way the answer you've been waiting for, naturally and suddenly, becomes obvious. You will have an "Aha" moment, or maybe a "Duh" moment—but either way, it's going to transform you, energize you and empower you.

The truth you're going to discover is this: there *is* a cure for compassion fatigue—there *is* an antidote for burnout—and the answer is not to take a step back, it's to take a step *forward*. When you use the tools and the insights in this book, they will allow you to create positive experiences of care for yourself and your patients, no matter what the circumstances. You will get back that confidence, that satisfaction, that personal sense of accomplishment that brought you into this profession in the first place. You just might become so accomplished at the process that you'll feel good all the time!

You opened this book because you are ready to bet the farm, hoping and praying that I know what I'm talking about, that I have the solution you know in your heart must exist, the answer you've been searching for but have yet to find. All of the concepts, tools and perspectives I have included here are designed with you in mind. They will lift you from the dark, heavy place of physical and emotional exhaustion, frustration or hopelessness you find yourself in today, and move you to higher ground, where you will live the high life for you will see what I see: you will see the future, and you will know (y)our future is bright.

"She Never Even Touched Me"

I have been practicing emergency medicine for almost thirty years, and I can say that the advances that American medicine has made in that time have been unprecedented and nothing less than spectacular. At the clinical level, I can do today, in a few hours' visit to the Emergency Department, what would have required a weeklong admission to the hospital back in the '80s. As a matter of fact, I can do more now than we even dreamed would be possible then.

Our modern technology-based medical system can do things today that my medical schoolteachers would never have thought possible. Our current system turns out novel treatments, impressive new surgeries and even seemingly miraculous cures each and every day. We can manage or control once fatal diseases and infections. We routinely transplant hearts, lungs, kidneys, livers and bone marrow. Advances in imaging with ever more sensitive ultrasound machines, CAT scanners, MRIs and PET scanners are changing the way we see and treat disease. We now have all sorts of implantable devices, pacemakers, defibrillators, neural stimulators, stents, knees, hips, ports and catheters. We can mobilize a heart cath team to open up a blocked coronary artery when you are having a heart attack, 24/7, almost anywhere in the country. We are sending cancers into remission every day.

Still, no one is satisfied. Many Americans now believe that modern medicine can, or should be able to, fix anything. With such high expectations, an aging population and high rates of disease, malpractice claims are at all-time highs as well. All of this costs money, so insurance rates are soaring, and the process of filing an insurance claim is getting more and more complicated. Hospitals and healthcare systems are struggling to get better patient outcomes, measure and report quality, minimize malpractice risk and bill effectively. Doctors and nurses are working harder than ever—and we're unhappier than ever.

In medicine, we rarely, if ever, hear that we did a good job, that we made the right diagnosis or significantly impacted the long-term outcome of our patients. The expectation is that doctors will bat a thousand. That we'll be right 100 percent of the time, be caring 100 percent of the time, that in any given situation we will know exactly what the right answer is and the right course of action should be. Anything less will result in a complaint or even a lawsuit. Perfection is expected, so that even when we make a miraculous save by participating in what we call a "Lazarus" case, patients—along with their families, our directors and our administrators—see it as us just doing our job. We rarely hear what we're doing right. Much of what we do is motivated by fear:

fear of being wrong, fear of the patient complaint, and the ultimate fear of a bad outcome and a lawsuit.

It's clear we are expected to bat a thousand; meanwhile, if we fall the slightest bit short—if we're batting .999—we get an earful. Even if we did everything correctly, if the patient complains, we are told, "You could have phrased what you said differently. You could have made a stronger effort to keep the patient and the family more informed as to what was going on. You could have communicated differently. You should have done better." I, for example, see roughly forty patients each shift. Fifteen shifts a month, roughly 600 patients. Over the course of four months, 4 out of 2,400 patients complained, and this is what I heard about. I was not told what a great job I did with the other 2,396 by anyone, This happens to every caregiver, every helper, every day in America. This is one of the reasons why there is so little satisfaction on our side of the stethoscope so much of the time.

When we look at problems within healthcare, or any public-service situation, we look only at the effects on the people being served. This keeps us from understanding the helpers' struggle, their stress, their pain and the issues they have to face in order to do their jobs. We focus solutions toward bettering results for the people they are serving—and rightly so; those people are victims in need. However, by forgetting the human factor on the caregivers' side of the equation, we make them out to be the villains instead of the heroes they really are and are expected to be.

The belief is that helpers should be born knowing what is best in these incredibly difficult, emotionally charged encounters and that they should be able to access this knowledge and act upon it in the heat of the moment—always and without exception. This may not be a conscious belief, but it is a powerful one, and it leads us into a situation where the healthcare worker is always critiqued in a Monday-morning-quarterback fashion. After the game has been played, everyone can see that the results were not optimal. Yet while those who are doing the critique are certain that things could have played out differently had the game been played better, they have no real or useful suggestions as to *how* the game could have been played better, and usually they're not putting on a uniform and getting in the game themselves. Our helpers, our care givers, are constantly left with the judgment that somehow what they did was not good enough. In a sense, they are constantly a failure, or at the very least *they are left feeling like no matter how perfectly they do their job, nothing really makes a difference.*

Of course, hospitals and healthcare systems are looking for ways to make things better, looking for ways to satisfy patients *and* attract good physicians and nurses, to achieve high levels of job satisfaction *and* employee engagement. Hospitals routinely survey their patients and post their satisfaction scores—when they are good. Patient satisfaction scores will soon be public information with the new HCAHPS surveys. Patient satisfaction scores will be tied to reimbursement. The government wants us to create a better "patient experience." Now that our president, the courts and our elected representatives have all had their say, implementation of the affordable care act will apply even more pressure for us to change, as it is crystal clear that Americans want something different from the goods and services we are currently delivering.

Paradoxically, and I believe this to be very true, these pressures and these changes have increased the quality of the physical care we deliver, but they've diminished the care we give in another way: they have taken our focus away from the patient and the energies contained in the interaction of giving and receiving care. We're forced to focus on the computerized chart, the ever-advancing technologies, quality-of-care measures, patient outcomes, evidence-based approaches, patient flow, cost effectiveness, efficiency and productivity, and none of those activities take place at the bedside.

Let's just look at one example: the use of electronic medical records, or the EMR. I recently spent some time in a hospital system that had not made the switch from paper. Although I thought I longed for the good ole days and fondly remembered my paper charts and my pen, I found that using paper is at least ten times harder than using an electronic medical record. Electronic medical records are of higher quality and more efficient, clearly better, especially for the patient. They ensure accuracy, avoid errors and are very thorough (as well as very billable)—in short, they improve the physical care we deliver to our patients.

Yet the computer is usually not at the bedside, and it's often far more efficient and more accurate to get the information we need to make decisions at the screen rather than taking the time to ask the patient questions, especially when, because of their circumstances, they have difficulty answering. So it often appears that the doctors and nurses are attending to the computer instead of attending to the patient, leaving the patient on the gurney wondering, *What's going on, why isn't anybody talking to me, why am I just lying here, doesn't anybody care?*

Even worse, when nursing and physician workstations are in plain view of patients and their families, they see us using the computers and phones, and they may even assume we are making social calls and surfing the Internet. Even though we are talking about them on the phone and researching them in the computer, they don't see that. So much of what we do in medicine today happens behind the scenes, away from the bedside, that it's no surprise our patients feel disconnected from us. Often patients will complain: *The doctor only spent a few minutes with me. He did not even talk to me. She never even touched me.*

No one is happy or satisfied within healthcare today, on either side of the stethoscope. This is the root of our problem. This is what I am writing about. This is why you are reading. There is no customer service guru or government official, no one from the entertainment or service industries who knows what it is like to be face to face with human pain and suffering the way we do. No one knows what it is like to tell a parent his or her child has died, except you. No one knows what it is like to hold a frail, elderly patient's hand as she passes away with no family present, but you. No one knows how to console a patient who's just been told he has cancer, better than you.

We can't wait for someone to save us. We, the givers of care, are in crisis. The situation has gone far beyond just happiness. Studies are showing us over and over again that this situation is making us emotionally and physically ill. We are all emotionally wounded. Call it compassion fatigue, call it burnout, call it secondary PTSD, but whatever you call it, the fact is clear that our humanity is being taken from us as a result of our working in healthcare today. We need to take responsibility for our crisis. Our very lives depend on it. This is our problem and only we, those of us who are at the bedside, in the trenches, with sick and hurting humans, can fix it. We must find a way to recover from compassion fatigue and connect with our patients again. No one else will do it for us; no one else can.

Our Heroic Journey Back to Humanity

Working in medicine is difficult and complicated, even on a good day. The pressures are intense and never-ending. Under circumstances like these, why would anyone want our jobs? Not for the money; there just isn't enough money. Those who do this for the money don't last long. We don't take these jobs for the healthcare benefits, the 401(k)s, the tuition reimbursement or the paid time off. We don't do these jobs because we have great hours or easy schedules.

You and I do this work because we want to care and to have our care make a difference. We want to be connected to something larger than ourselves, to a mission to ease pain and suffering in our world. We do these jobs because we want to be connected to a group of people who want the same thing. We do these jobs so that at the end of the day we can say we matter and we are doing the important work of helping others.

When it is all said and done, what do we, the people at the bedside, want? We want to be someone's hero. What is so great about this is that our patients want and desperately need someone to be their hero too. Our patients want us to step out of the ordinary, to think outside the box, to color outside the lines. Our patients want us to be *extra*-ordinary. Our patients want to feel our care; they want us to make a difference for them. Our desires on both sides of the stethoscope are the same.

My job is to provide you with the **one and only real solution** that will allow you to create true satisfaction on both sides of the stethoscope—for yourself, those you work with and those you care for. You can apply this solution to absolutely any clinical environment and it will always produce the desired result. This solution works, and it works right now. It worked yesterday and I can guarantee that it will work tomorrow. In the chapters ahead, I will give you the reasons why it works, show you how I made it work for me and give you the tools to make it work for you.

The book you are holding in your hands right now is a road map—well, more like a treasure map—that leads you back from burnout, back to the satisfaction you hunger for in your career and in your life. You'll learn how you can, simply through the care you give to another, create that satisfaction, nurture it and recreate it as often as you need to. This is information you won't find anywhere else, not in other books, not in medical school or nursing school—there's no course called Caring 101—and certainly not in your daily experience, if your daily experience is anything like mine used to be. This is a new path, and we are pathfinders.

Together you and I are going on a journey of our own—a quest to find out how to create satisfaction on both sides of the stethoscope. Have you heard of a quantum leap? Well, we are going to take a giant leap to a new level of satisfaction and a new level of care, what I call the quantum level, that level of reality where the science of quantum mechanics applies. This is where true fulfillment can be created. Nothing around you has to change, and yet you will change, and, mysteriously, everything and everyone around you will change too. You will become the model—and the cause—of the change you want to see in your world.

Once you have walked all the steps on your own healthcare hero's journey, you will be amazed to discover that you are fully involved in and enthusiastic about your work. You will be happier and more energetic, more resilient, more innovative and a better problem solver. You will feel more connected and more concerned about the health of your patients and your peers. You will once again be sure that you are doing meaningful work in the world. You will not waste so much time daydreaming about winning the lottery or wondering what else you could do for a living.

It's a rather short journey, a day trip really. Even better, it's not all rocket science. We'll start by agreeing that all we want is to feel good. Next we will look at the things that stand in the way of our feeling good. Then we will see what we need to get over those barriers. I'll show you what I have discovered about care, what stops us from caring and how we can bring true care back into everything we do.

The process is simple enough and there are only seven steps. To make them easier to remember and use in real time while at the patient's bedside—or even at the family dinner table—we will use the mnemonic "**R.E.F.L.E.C.T.**" First we will **Remember** why we came here to healthcare in the first place, and we will reconnect with our pure and simple desire to care, to make things better, to help and to make a difference. Next we will realize that it's up to us to **Earn** our own satisfaction: no one can give satisfaction to you, only you can create the satisfaction you crave. Next I will illustrate how you can recalculate the transaction of care and **Formulate** your plan for it. Then I'll show you how we will reframe our interaction with our patient when we **Look** to see if we are the cause or the effect inside the patient encounter. Soon we will **Evaluate** our situation to see if our care is making a difference for our patient and making us feel good; if it's not, then we will start the process again as we **Circle back** to the beginning. Finally we will restore and renew ourselves by learning to **Take care** of ourselves, giving us new power to transcend our present limitations so that we are ready to face a new day in a new way.

Once inside the journey, we will see what satisfaction really is, where it comes from and how it can be achieved. I'll give you the magic bullet I call the **TIME OUT** tool—the one and only weapon you will ever need to slay any dragon—and show you how to use it in the clinical situations we encounter over and over again so that when one of them pops up, you already have the framework for a solution. And I'll teach you the **Perfect Equation**, the formula that will always enable you to create quantum satisfaction, not only for yourself but for your patient as well. The Perfect Equation is foolproof and flawless. It never fails, unless you don't truly want to care.

You already do the impossible and the heroic each and every day. I am here to reconnect you to your purpose, your initial desire to help, to relight your fire—and show you how to keep the fire burning each and every day. If you embrace what I am sharing with you, take it to heart and use it wisely, you will once again be reunited with your passion to care for others. This passion will get you out of bed in the morning, excited and ready to spend the day caring for others at work. The people you work with will be genuinely happy to see you and work alongside you.

Today is the day everything begins to change for you, so get ready! I am going to help you to reignite your passion and transform your care so that it makes a difference and saves the day. I'm going to help you become the modern day hero of healthcare you were always destined to be.

Regardless of your circumstances, when you leave home for work, you will look in the mirror and like what you see. Better yet, when you return home at the end of your incredible day, you can look into the same mirror and say, *What I did today mattered. Today was a good day.*

Chapter 1

Care in Crisis

Not so long ago, in the middle of a long, cold, grey winter in Ohio, I was working the night shift in the emergency department of a suburban/urban hospital. We were open to all squad traffic, and we were a chest pain center as well as a level II trauma center. We had inpatient psychiatry and pediatrics. This was a really busy place.

No one feels good this time of year here. People tend to fall victim to the flu, strep throat, pneumonia, bronchitis and the like. Shoveling snow can bring on the "big one," and depressed patients feel worse than ever. People slip on the ice and break all sorts of bones. Emergency departments are always busy and hospitals are always full, no room at the inn, so to speak.

This was an exceptionally busy and chaotic night; patients had been waiting a long time to get back into beds from the waiting room. These patients were frustrated and angry, especially when we brought back the chest pain in front of the twisted ankle. No matter who you are, when you come to the emergency department for care, you feel yours is the biggest emergency and deserves top priority. And this night I was the lone physician on duty, without any residents to train or mid-level providers to help me.

I was passionate about being a doctor, but I was even more passionate about being an emergency physician. I so LOVE the EMERGENCY. Caring for cases that aren't emergencies can be frustrating, especially when the patient is needy or demanding. But inside the emergency, the angel of death is in the room. The pressure is intense, yet there is a calm, a peace, like being in the eye of the storm. Everything becomes crystal clear to me, and the problems and priorities are obvious. I know exactly what needs to be done and the order in which in needs to be done.

But more than anything else, the real emergency is where what I do, the training that I have, the skills I have learned, the knowledge that I have fought to learn and retain, really matters. Where what I do matters most. Where I have the capacity and the ability to make the biggest impact, make the biggest change, in all of medicine. Where what I do—the tests I order and the treatments or medicines I give, the specialists and sub-specialists I involve—in those first few minutes or seconds of my encounter with the patient (who is clearly in desperate need of my help, my talents, my care) will, if done properly, make all the difference in the world. Helping others inside the emergency was my purpose, my reason for living, and my salvation.

Beelzebub in the Parking Lot

I had always wanted to be a doctor. As soon as I could walk, I wanted to be a doctor. My mom had pictures of me bandaging up all the dogs in the neighborhood. High school was to get into college, college was to get into medical school, medical school was to get into residency and residency would give me board certification as an emergency physician. A dream come true. I gave my childhood, my adolescence and all my early adult years to that dream. It sustained me, nurtured me, supported me and held me.

Then, shortly after I finished my internship, in the very beginning of my practice of medicine, during my first year as an attending physician, something happened. I was diagnosed with testicular cancer. I had some surgery and some other treatments, and I did well. No big deal. I went on with my life and my career. Just when things seemed to be moving in the right direction and my life was starting to look pretty good, out of the blue it seemed, something happened again, and I was devastated. My soul screamed, "Not cancer! Not again! No, not now!" If my life ended now, it would be a tragedy, a wasted life. I had yet to leave my mark.

I was thirty-eight years old, and this time the cancer was worse, and it had spread. The doctors were telling me I very possibly might die, even with treatment. While I had some of the very best and most talented and compassionate physicians and surgeons, I decided to leave no stone unturned. I saw shamans, psychologists and energy workers as well. I looked at the psycho-spiritual causes of my cancer and did visualizations and meditations. Finally, I had the mutilating surgery and the poisonous chemotherapy and it was awful. Somehow, by the grace of God, I managed to get through the cancer for a second time.

My second brush against cancer definitely changed me. I was a different person afterwards. I felt as if I had been awakened spiritually. I realized that there was more to life. I had been given another chance at life and I wasn't planning on wasting this one. This time, not only was I going to get it all, I was going to "get it all" right.

Once I had recuperated physically, I went on a mission to get all the things I thought I needed to have a great life and, above all, be happy. I set out to get it all: the best job, a gorgeous spouse, the best house in the best neighborhood, the best dog, no, I wanted two great dogs, the best car, no, I needed two cars, one SUV to get to the hospital no matter rain, sleet, snow or ice and a really sharp, cool, fast, hot convertible Mustang. I was bound and determined to have the best of everything.

Most important of all, I was going to get back on the other side of the stethoscope. I loved the idea of being a doctor! I had been living the dream, and when the cancer took that away from me, I was lost. The idea of giving a second chance to others, as my doctors had done for me twice already, was the one thing that really set me on fire.

Soon enough, I was working harder than ever to get all those things I thought I needed to make my life significant and meaningful "now", and I do mean right now. Patience has never been my strong suit. In retrospect, the next ten years of my life passed quickly.

I was immersed in the process. I was healthy and free of disease. I was in remission, dare I say, cured! I had crafted a new life. In those ten years I really did get it all, everything I wanted, including some awesome vacations—and, sadly, I realized that I had never felt emptier. I had done everything I felt I was supposed to do, yet something was wrong. It seemed to me that my recipe for success was missing a key ingredient.

You see, to get all this stuff I thought I needed to be successful in life, especially after my second diagnosis of cancer, I was working harder than ever as an emergency-department doctor and finding myself coming up short at the end of each work day, exhausted and frustrated. Things had gotten much more difficult in the ten years that had passed since I returned to work.

First, there was the malpractice crisis, which, in a nutshell, ate up almost all of the physician group's revenue, so our salaries fell. Then, out of the blue, the nursing shortage hit. All of those seasoned, compassionate nurses seemed to disappear, and when (or if) they were replaced, they were replaced with brand-new grads who had no clinical experience except for their orientation to the ED. The Certified Emergency Nurse became an extinct species. Finally, the economy in the area went belly-up as the two largest employers closed the plants and took the manufacturing jobs elsewhere. .

As a result, although the physicians and the physician assistants remained the same, almost all of the nurses disappeared, so that there was little if any experienced nursing on the floor at any given time. And because many in the community lost their health insurance when the plants closed, the numbers presenting to the emergency department for care went up dramatically. Often, now, our patients were underinsured or flat-out uninsured. Many had no family doctor, no other way to seek care at all.

All of this increased the pressure in the emergency department dramatically. We were now preoccupied with overcrowding and ambulance diversion. We were talking about productivity scores and patient satisfaction scores, core measures and best practices. Wait times were up and "lengths of stay" were getting longer. And no matter how hard I worked, it never seemed to get easier, only harder. Each night when I arrived, there would be double digits waiting in triage, 20, 25, 33 . . . and I would jump right in and work as hard and fast as possible. My documentation suffered because of the acuity and volume, so my dictations were returned to me for clarification. I was constantly being distracted from tasks at hand because the new-grad nurses had questions. Many times there would be a line of nurses waiting to ask questions that I felt that they should already know the answers to. I was rapidly growing tired of teaching them everything they needed to know to be excellent Emergency Department nurses, only to have them desert me for the first day-shift position available so that I would have to teach another new grad everything, all over again.

Each and every night that I walked into that department, I felt terrified that I would not be enough to handle the situation(s). I was hypervigilant, worried that somewhere in the department, in the double digits in triage that I had not seen yet, there was an unrecognized sick one who might deteriorate rapidly or even die in the lobby. I am not kidding! I worried that if there was a sick baby, or a patient with an unusual presentation of a serious problem, this would go unrecognized, and the potential for death in the lobby was real and ever-present. I worried that I would not be fast enough, smart enough, clever enough or powerful enough to keep something bad from happening to any of my patients. It literally felt like the Angel of Death had a decked-out Winnebago, flames on the side and everything, parked just beyond the ambulance bay. Anytime Beelzebub was falling short on his "quota" he could just snag a couple from our poorly defended lobby.

A Very Deep Hole

I was not about to let death in the lobby happen—ever! Here is what I did to push that system to its limits—and I mean to the very edge of what was possible. I would become the fastest night-shift emergency-room doctor ever in the history of modern medicine. No, in the history of humankind. I would be the best clinician. I would develop my sense of smell to the point that I could smell which patient was the sickest just by holding their chart in my hand. I would grow eyes in the back of my head so that I could see all of the accidents that were waiting to happen and intervene before anything went wrong.

I felt like one of those little ducks that you see at the county fair, moving across the game trailer slowly, where the idea is to shoot one with a gun and knock it over for a prize. I felt like a sitting duck because in that malpractice climate, one unexpected death or bad case could make any one of us uninsurable; in effect, we stood to lose our ability to practice medicine. All I wanted was to find the sickest of the sick in the midst of the sea of those looking for care so that I could hold onto my license.

My plan was to move the patients through the department as fast as I could. My goal was to empty out the lobby, see every patient for myself, to make certain that no one died because someone else did not recognize how sick they were or did not realize how quickly their condition could deteriorate. I felt sort of like a glorified traffic cop. I wanted to make certain that the nurses, the PAs, the patients and the ambulances were all working with me to keep all the patients moving out a door—the door that led to the elevators and the inpatient beds or the door that led to the parking lot and home.

Either door was okay with me, just so long as they kept moving out of our department. That way if something sick came into the lobby or if a squad came in with something critical, we would have the space and the resources so that I could give "it"—well, actually, "them"—my undivided attention. I did not realize it at the time, but I was systematically objectifying my patients, turning them in to caricatures of their disease or situation. Much easier to work with them this way, like chess pieces on a board.

I needed the staff to work hard for me, so with them I was friendly, gregarious and helpful most of the time. I told jokes to lighten the mood. I played music to drown out the chaos. Sometimes I would sing along. But I was spending less and less time at the bedside with my patients, keeping my "professional" distance. I would put on my plastic, emotionless, politically correct face and wear it with an incredibly snug fit, especially when I was in a patient room or dealing with family members. There was absolutely no way I would let these two groups see the sheer terror in my eyes. No way they were gonna see me sweat. I would be nothing but professional, detached and clinical. I developed an air that bordered on arrogance.

"They don't pay me to smile, ma'am. Sir, I am not paid to hold your hand. My job is to do the history and physical exam, complete a diagnostic evaluation and provide you with a treatment plan. Excuse me, miss, just the facts, nothing else, I am extremely busy and there are many other patients who need my help. I am sorry you had to wait so long to get into a room, but complaining to me about the wait is useless and will only cause other patients to wait longer. Here is the number of the hospital administrator. Call them tomorrow and complain to them. They get paid to listen to your complaints about the care you receive here; I don't. So if you don't mind, let us begin. Why are you here today?"

Not surprisingly, the number of patient complaints I was receiving was on the rise and my patient satisfaction scores were in the toilet. The patients complained that I seemed rushed, distracted, uncaring or even downright rude. I counter-complained to the other ED physicians I worked with, and I complained very loudly to our ED Physician Director: "Patients are waiting in the lobby four and five hours to get into rooms—how can they possibly be satisfied? I have no control over that. I am doing my best. I can't work any harder. No other physician except the one working nights has these challenges."

Also not surprisingly, the partner doctors I worked with in the emergency department started to grow weary of this incessant complaining. They no longer took me seriously; they wanted to know, did I want cheese with my whine? While I was not the only one complaining, I was the one complaining most loudly and most often. Also, because I was jovial, told jokes and was friendly with the nurses, while at the same time the patients were saying I didn't seem to care, my partners started to feel that I did not take my job seriously.

At one of my performance evaluations with our director, I was told to be more professional, not to sing or tell jokes. *Don't be friendly with the staff. Remember the nurses are not your friends. Instead of telling jokes, spend more time in the patients' rooms, explaining their tests and treatments.* I countered, "Are you serious? I don't have the time to go to the bathroom, let alone sit down in a patient's room. You have no idea what is really going on in this department. Some director you are!"

The thing saving me was that I was a good doctor and I was good at taking care of patients, medically speaking. No malpractice claims or medical complaints or cases falling out for peer review. But in every other respect I had dug a very deep hole for myself. I hated going to work. I dreaded just getting into the car to drive there.

Are you getting a sense of the sort of results my plan was yielding me? Let me tell you about a grandfather who came with his young daughter and his grandson. This man's grandson was having a severe asthma attack. The child was really struggling to breathe, so he was placed in a room very close to my desk, which was in plain view of the entire department near the ambulance entrance. Grandpa, as it turned out, was retired from a position as an efficiency expert with a corporate giant. He apparently did not like my rushed, detached and professional demeanor with his daughter and grandson. He proceeded to ask the nurse for a pen and paper. He peered at me—no, he stared a hole in my back—as he looked from outside the curtain, watching my every move.

While I thought he was just angry and fuming, he was actually very busy with a project of his own. Since his grandson was on the "Asthma Care Path," he had to wait for two hours after a breathing treatment to be reassessed so that we could determine if he could be discharged or would need to be admitted to the hospital. His grandson was in the department, in the room next to my desk, for just about seven hours. The entire time, his grandpa got angrier and angrier.

The man's grandson did well and was ultimately discharged home, feeling better after his dramatic presentation and his severe difficulty breathing. His grandfather was not appreciative or thankful at all, and he took direct aim at me. What had he been doing the entire time he was in the emergency department? Well, it obviously wasn't consoling his grandson or his daughter. He was timing me. He, being an efficiency expert, knowing nothing about medicine, thought that I was doing everything all wrong. He sent a scathing letter to administration about what an incompetent and inefficient quack I was. He did not list one complaint about the medical care his grandson received. But he was quick to tell administration that I should be fired.

Why? Because in the seven or so hours that he was observing me, he documented that I spent X number of minutes on the phone (obviously making personal calls). X number of minutes "playing" on the computer, obviously surfing the web for pleasure. X number of minutes interacting directly with the nurses, obviously making small talk and telling jokes, as I was smiling and laughing. And the list continued.

Worse yet, when I was called on the carpet because of this letter, I was told I should not do those things. It did not seem to matter that I was using the computer for patient care, and that the phone calls were either calls to the dictation system to dictate charts or calls to other physicians to secure follow-up or get patients admitted. The time I spent interacting with nurses was to give them direction regarding patient care and patient flow. None of that mattered. I was told that perception is reality, and I made it look too easy, like I was having fun even, and that was unacceptable.

There is nothing more frustrating for me than working long hours, working hard, and being told that your patients are not happy with you and that you—worst of all—are uncaring. It hurt me deeply when I was accused of not caring. After all, my whole plan was to keep them all safe from the angel of death. It did not matter that the medical care that I delivered was safe, conservative and sound. The patients were not complaining about the medicine they got from me. They were complaining about my bedside manner. They saw me as cold-hearted. They felt that I did not care.

Why was I practicing this way? I was already overwhelmed. I was doing exactly what I had been told in medical school—don't get too close to my patients, don't get involved, you will lose your objectivity, you won't be able to handle their pain, it will consume you and destroy you. I wanted to be fast, efficient, accurate. There was nothing worse for my plan than to get caught up in a patient's room, at the bedside, getting involved and all of that stuff. My feeling was that the broken "system" was the reason that I could not get any fulfillment or satisfaction and that my patients could not feel my care.

I always managed to get that broken system to give my patients what they needed, medically speaking, although it may not necessarily have been what they wanted. Then that dreadful day came when the final straw was delivered that broke this doctor's back.

Chapter 2

When Cows Fly

One day I had a patient who needed surgery to repair the ligaments in her dislocated elbow. Surgery was the only solution; no matter how many times I reduced it manually, it would not stay in place. But when I called the orthopedic doctor on call, he said that he could not care for her because he had a whole day of surgeries booked. He would not make himself available, even though he was on call and, by law, had to care for this patient no matter what. I went up the chain of command and got no support. After hours of phone calls, I was finally able to get another orthopedic doctor to care for this patient as a personal favor to me.

I'd had problems with this particular on-call doctor since our very first meeting. He thought I was incompetent and poorly trained. I thought he was arrogant and money-hungry and suffered from severe small-man syndrome. The two of us always clashed. Did he refuse to give my patient surgery just because of our interpersonal difficulties? No, I was convinced he did not care for her just because it was inconvenient for him. That was the straw that broke the camel's back. I could not get this patient what she needed, surgery, and if I can't get my patients what they need, then I can't do my job. Once I left the hospital that day, I found the courage to quit.

What was I thinking when I quit? I felt misunderstood and wrongly judged. How could anybody really believe for one second that I did not care? How could administration even take that letter from the efficiency grandpa seriously? How could an on-call specialist refuse to care for a patient and *not* get in trouble? I was thinking when I quit that nobody cared except me, and that my biggest problem, in fact, was that I cared too much!

So now what? Jobless and in debt up to my eyeballs, I clearly had no plan. I did not want to work clinically any longer, but the only thing I knew was medicine. I had given my whole life to medicine. What else could I do? What else did spending twenty-plus years in a room full of a hundred angry complainers qualify me to do? I decided to take some time off and figure it all out.

What had happened to me that morning that I had such a hard time getting my patient the surgery she needed? No one supported me. No one seemed to care—except for one person, the orthopedic surgeon who stepped up to the plate to care for this patient. He didn't do it because he had to; he did it because he sensed my frustration and he wanted to help. I realized that what had happened was that someone else finally cared for me, and as a result, he cared for my patient.

Up to this point, I'd felt like I was the only one who really cared. Everything I was doing came from my desire to care for the patients, keep them safe, get them what they needed. In my mind, I was doing my very best to make a broken system work. I thought I had to move quickly and be cut-and-dried with my patients so that I could save the life of that one patient in the lobby whose condition might go unrecognized. I made sure my patients got taken care of, always. It might not have looked or felt the way they wanted it to look or feel, they may not have gotten what they wanted, but they always got what I felt they needed. **It hurt me deeply when they complained that I did not care**. Their conclusions about me seemed senseless. To me it wasn't that I never cared, it was that I cared too much. (It would be much later that I would learn that the truth was something else altogether—I was confused about what care really was.)

I did not see myself as cold and heartless, but when I started to think back on that case, I realized that I couldn't remember the woman's name, the color of her eyes, her skin or her hair color or even the way she had injured herself. I could not remember who was with her. I could remember almost nothing about her except which room she was in, what medications I gave her, what her x-rays looked like and who it was that finally decided to step up to the plate and take her to the operating room for her surgery. What did that tell me about myself?

What I started to realize was that, while I saw the one orthopedic doctor as an ass who did not care, he was just mirroring back to me the fact that **I was being an ass to my patients almost all the time. I had been trying to survive by not connecting personally** with my patients, focusing on their physical needs alone, not caring for them emotionally or spiritually, wearing my plastic emotionless face, being disconnected and clinical and—I thought—professional. I had believed that I was doing my very best, but that was not the me I wanted to be. It was *keeping* me from being the best version of myself, the doctor I truly aspired to be.

During my time off, without working clinically, I'd realized that being a doctor was not just what I did for a living, but actually *who I was*. I liked taking care of people, and more than anything else I loved saving seriously sick or injured patients, giving them another chance at life. I loved wrestling with the angel of death, against the clock, against all odds; I loved being the very best at what I did, knowing what to do and how to do it. I loved saving lives! I could not imagine my own life without being able to do that.

It was clearly time for me to step back into the fire. It was time for me to go back to work. And this time it was going to be different. This time I was going to connect the dots. I was going to get my patients what they needed physically, and I wasn't going to stop there. I was going to spend more time at the bedside and I was going to see to it that they were satisfied with everything that I was working so hard to do for them. This time, when I stepped onto the floor, I was going to get it right.

I decided that no matter how high the bullshit level was, how bad the environment might be, I would have to put up with it and find new ways to cope with it. I reconnected with my initial and original desire to care, to make a difference, to change things and save the day for my patients, and I set out in search of a new job. I found one, and initially it was great. But, after a while, the shine began to tarnish and many of the same old dragons and demons started to show up. I found myself wrestling with the same problems and feelings again—feelings of being taken for granted, unappreciated, overtaxed, overwhelmed.

Which brings us to that cold, grey night in Northeast Ohio when something very big happened. I didn't realize it at the time—it took much longer—but that night would change the way I thought about medicine, and about myself, forever.

The Night of the Purple Cows

The volume of patients who came through our ED every night and the complexities of caring for them would put pressure on anyone, under the best of circumstances. Because our patients often don't have the capacity to tell us even what medications they're taking, the sheer amount of research and number of phone calls it takes to attend to just one person can be overwhelming. And with the ED understaffed—me essentially alone on the job—these were not the best of circumstances. My feelings of angst and frustration were really starting to boil up into my mind when I picked up a chart where the chief complaint said simply, "PSYCH EVAL. Stopped taking psych meds one or two months ago, ok right now, but having trouble with increased agitation."

I went into the psych room to see a very large man with blond hair, six foot one and 320 pounds, sitting there sweating, disheveled and anxious in gym shorts and a long-sleeved button-down shirt hanging open. "Hello," I said to him. "How can I help you?"

He turned to me, clearly agitated, yet somehow able to look at me with that desperate gleam of hope in his eye, hope that I just might be able to help. "Please, doctor!" he cried. "You've got to stop these flying purple cows from trying to have sex with me."

What was my first thought? I have to be honest: it was not about caring for him, it was not about helping him. My first feelings for him were more like exasperation that he was not caring for himself, not taking his meds, that the system was broken, that his case manager dropped the ball. I was frustrated that he was even here, in the emergency department, when all he needed to do was take his medicine.

In other words, my first thought was about me. *Great, just what I need*, I thought. *The department is busy and the patients are sick, there are double digits out in the waiting room, and now I have an actively hallucinating crazy man to take care of. Just freaking great! Does it ever end?*

Thinking back, I don't remember if I even answered him. I believe I just looked down at the dirty floor and walked out of his room. I do remember quickly putting some orders in for him and moving on, racing against the clock to see all the patients who were already in rooms so that I could move them through the process. I was busy running the department, checking to see whose test results were back, who should be feeling better after the treatments I had ordered, who was ready to be discharged and who I needed to call to get another patient admitted, and intermittently catching up on my paper charting at the desk, when all of a sudden I heard some loud commotion. It seemed to be coming from the psych room. I went to investigate and found this giant of a crazy man in the hallway outside the psych rooms, near the med station, beating the crap out of one of my medics.

I tried to break it up and all of a sudden I was on the floor, in a full nelson, with this larger-than-life enraged psychotic man on top of me, all red in the face and wide-eyed, choking me, trying to kill me! He wants me dead! Talk about shock and awe! I started turning purple in the face myself as I shouted orders for medicine from underneath his chokehold. The narrow hallway where he lay on top of me was filling up with people—two ambulance crews who happened to be in the department dropping off patients, all of my ED staff, the entire security department, could not get the giant blond off me. Someone called 911 and now there were six officers from the local police force, complete with tazers—all trying to figure out a way to get control of the situation—but he only choked me harder.

Inside any emergency, time seems to stand still, and seconds seem like hours, and this went on for what seems like an unbelievable amount of time. In reality, I was in this guy's chokehold for something like 45 minutes—during which the entire emergency department ground to a halt. "Get this guy off of me!" I screamed as patients and their families peeked out from behind their curtains to see the spectacle. But to me it was deadly serious: I thought I might actually die here on the dirty emergency department floor. *Is this it?* I wondered. God's sick cruel joke, my life ends in tragedy, headlines read: *Doctor killed by crazy patient.*

I don't remember exactly how they loosened his hold on me, how I wiggled out from under him, but I do now appreciate the wisdom of my residency training: never wear a tie in the emergency department. I believe that it was adrenalin and brute force, coupled with their desire to help me and protect the patient that allowed the situation to resolve. I had been shouting orders for sedatives, and these were probably starting to take effect too. The bottom line is that I am here and able to tell the story. Eventually, we were able to get the man back into his room and strap him in a bed.

Then it was back to the business of managing patient flow and running the emergency department. Imagine me standing up, walking away, while everyone else was getting him back to his room and strapping him down. Out of breath, sweating, clothes torn, and the only doctor. No time for recovery for me; more patients had checked in through triage, and the patients already in the department could see that the entertainment was over and they wanted their diagnosis and disposition. Squads had brought patients who could not breathe into our only open beds. No time to think about what had just happened. I had to get busy being the doctor.

Hours later, I had finally managed to get everyone seen, no one was waiting, everyone was in the process of receiving care or undergoing their diagnostic evaluations. Most of the patients who'd been there during the "show" had been discharged or admitted. Finally, maybe a deep breath. I was sitting at my desk, getting to some paperwork at last, when Joe appeared, frantic. Now, Joe and frantic don't belong in the same sentence; you see, Joe is one of the best ED and charge nurses I have ever worked with. He pounded on my countertop.

Bam bam. "Damn it, Doc, come on," he said. "He's blue and he's not breathing." Together we rushed back toward the psych room. "I was just in here less than two minutes ago," Joe was saying. "He tried to bite me, and when he couldn't, he spit in my face instead."

In his room, the large man troubled by purple cows lay there lifeless, strapped with leather to the bed. In seconds the restraints came off, we started CPR, I intubated him, and then we transferred him to another cart and rushed him into the trauma bay. Soon we had a pulse and a blood pressure, but he needed the ventilator—he was not breathing on his own, and his pupils were fixed and dilated. Neurologically speaking, he was unresponsive. We sent him up to the ICU and I and my staff once again went back to work, as if the work of trying to resuscitate a human being is not work.

Later that morning, after the shift was over and I was already home trying to fall asleep, I got the dreaded call that the morbidly obese blond-haired crazy man whom flying purple cows found so irresistible, the crazy man who tried to kill me, had died.

I had been praying so hard that he would recover, and this call hit me really hard. The earth shook. I felt sick. I suddenly was afraid that I would be blamed for his death. Somehow, they would make this my fault. Had I done something wrong? Did I miss something?

I was afraid—no, that is not strong enough—I was *terrified* that my career was over. I was certain there would be a malpractice case. I believed that I had come to a dead end; I felt like Thelma and wondered, where is Louise? My world as I knew it had come to an end. I did not know how I would find the strength to put on my white coat and get behind a stethoscope again.

The Truth about Care

There was no sleeping after receiving that call. I had to find a way to get myself showered, shaved, dressed and to the hospital to drive that stethoscope from room to room to say hello to and care for patients. I had to face the staff I'd worked with the very night before, who'd helped me care for the man, who'd pulled the man off of me, who'd gotten calls themselves earlier in the day with the news that he'd passed away.

It's not that none of my patients had ever died before. Sometimes, even when everything goes perfectly right, patients die. This was different. Exactly how it was different is tough to articulate, but let's just say that it totally consumed me. This man's death, less than twenty-four hours after he had tried to kill me with his bare hands, well, it shook me to the core of my being.

The authorities were notified, of course. Everybody and their brother investigated the unexpected death, and until the statute of limitations ran out—two years—I crossed my fingers, soul-searched and prayed. But there was nothing to find—everything had been done right. There were no fines, no penalties and no malpractice case, not even a deposition. Still, even though no one could find anything wrong with my clinical performance the night of what we dubbed "The Happening," I experienced lots of pain, lots of guilt and lots of fear. In all the work I have done with therapists and healers, I have learned that guilt, fear and pain are always signs telling us to look deeper to find the root of the problem, for only then can the solution emerge. For two years, I relived that night over and over again in my heart and in my mind, looking for answers.

Why did I feel so emotional about this case? Was it because he'd tried to kill me? Although some of my patients have been so angry they could not say the word *doctor* without putting the F word in front of it, no one had ever really tried to kill me before. That had to be the reason, right? No, that wasn't it. It just wasn't.

I thought and thought about what I could have done differently that night I was nearly strangled to death on the dirty emergency-room floor. And I realized that although I hadn't done anything medically or professionally wrong, something else I hadn't done was connect with, or even really care for, this poor man. What did I do when I walked into that room and said hello as he begged me to help him? At that moment, even though his illness had a stranglehold on his sanity, he managed to reach out. I did not return the favor. I did not acknowledge his suffering. I did not connect to him. I stayed inside myself. I didn't feel for him; I didn't really see him. All I cared about, really, even while I was doing my very best at my job, was me: how many more patients were waiting to see *me*, how *I* was going to make it through my shift. Even when I heard that he had died, my first thoughts were about me. *Oh my God, my career is over. My life is over. He wins. He's killed me after all.*

Where had I seen this piece of me before in my clinical life? The all-business, just-the-facts-ma'am, it's busy here and I have other patients to tend to—*that* Frank Gabrin? It was not that long ago. Remember the job I quit because the orthopedic surgeon was such a jerk? That is where I had seen that version of me before. At first I had thought I was quitting because the working environment was intolerable and that I was a victim at work, that in reality no one cared but me. "They" did not care; "they" were assholes. Back then I thought I had figured out what I needed to learn about care myself. I thought I had turned over a new leaf with my resolution to put aside my plastic professional face and spend time at the bedside. Yet here I was again, in a different job, in a different clinical situation, but back in that same familiar place, doing the same things. Only this time, someone had died.

This discovery reverberated with my initial desire to care, to make a difference, to change the world and save the day. Because I had not truly cared for this man, **I'd missed my opportunity to get what I really wanted**: the feeling that comes from connecting with a patient, feeling empathy for them and generating compassion for them. None of that requires a stethoscope, a medicine, an IV, a needle or an X-ray. What a revelation. **I was the reason I felt bad**.

When I took the time off between jobs, I had realized how much I missed taking care of people. I realized that the person I was being in that environment was not the person I wanted to be.

Now, with the added clarity that the purple cows had brought my way, I began to see that I wasn't a victim of the broken system, the callous administrators, the government, the patients or the other doctors. My own misconceptions, attitudes and beliefs, my personal and professional baggage, my personal and professional defenses were the things that kept me from truly caring, truly connecting with my patients. Now I could clearly see that connecting with my patients was something that I wanted, more than anything. Something that I needed personally to feel good about who I am and what I do! But wait, we were taught, no, we were warned not to get too close. Getting too close would overwhelm us. Getting too close would cause us to lose our objectivity. Getting too close would make it impossible for us to make good decisions. No wonder I felt confused and conflicted.

But now, in this pivotal case, where purple cows were flying through the air, torturing my patient and demanding sex from him, if I had really made the effort to connect with him, to care about him, he might have felt it on some level and been reassured rather than frightened. Maybe the outcome would have been, well, let's say, different. Or maybe it would have been no different. The truth is that I will never know, but what I know now is that I will always feel bad about this encounter for one reason and one reason alone: I was uncaring. That was what haunted me, not the fact of the man's passing.

Realizing that, although I had spent over twenty years caring for others, **I really did not know what care was, and I did not know how to care**—it shook me, it spooked me, it rocked my world. Yeah, I knew how to examine patients, order tests, read X-rays and EKGs, order medicines, interpret results, involve the appropriate specialists and get my patients what they needed physically, but I did not connect on a personal level with them most of the time. I did not feel their pain, empathize with them, reassure them or cry with them when nothing else could be done. Perhaps this is why there are tears in my eyes as I type these very words. **I really did not know what care was then, so how could I have known how to care?**

Chapter 3

What Care Is

Hindsight is 20/20, and thank God for that, because without it, I would not be the doctor or the man I am today. And honestly and truly I can finally say that today I am proud of who I am because I care, I make a difference, I change the world and I save the day. This is what is important to me and this is what I do. The only way I or anyone else can do this is by making that personal connection, empathizing with our patients and feeling their pain. Most importantly however, once we are connected to them and their pain, we must find a way to move from empathy to feeling real compassion for them. That is how we can truly care for them. That is also how we make them feel better, but more than anything else, turning on our own compassion is what makes us feel better; feel good about who we are and what we are doing.

Personally, I—like many of the smart adults I work with in the hospital—have problems with relationships. (Relationships are challenging for people suffering from compassion fatigue and burnout—remember the Surgeon General's warning at the beginning of the book!) Yet there is nothing truly worthwhile in this life that does not come through our connection to others. I had to do a lot, and I do mean a lot, of research and read a lot of books to figure this out for myself, because we certainly aren't taught this in medical school or on the job. Just the opposite: our own medical and nursing literature tells us that compassion fatigue is the direct and inevitable result of caring for patients who are in significant emotional pain and physical distress. We are told over and over again to stay detached—not to connect with our patients, to get friendly with them, to get too close to them, because this will remove our objectivity, cloud our judgment and make it impossible for us to make good clinical decisions. We are taught to believe that feeling the pain of our patients will consume and destroy us.

Just so you know, they really did teach us this. You will most commonly find this wisdom imbedded in our textbooks for nursing, medicine and allied health in the sections where you find the discussions of professionalism. What's more, everyone I have asked about this idea of professional detachment, and the resulting objectivity it affords us, believes the notion to be true. There's even a recent study telling us that too much empathy impedes the delivery of quality medical care—so now it appears that they are telling us to distance ourselves even further, injecting even more fear with the notion that without that distance, we will actually make mistakes.

The industry wants us to smile but remain emotionally disconnected—to put on that plastic professional face and keep our professional distance. And this "disconnect" between "personal" and "professional" pervades all of medicine. But the connection that's absent here—the connection to both our patient and our original pure, uncorrupted, simple desire to care—is the missing ingredient we are all looking for. It is the missing piece of the puzzle. The truth they didn't teach us in medical or nursing school is this: it's not when we care too much that we burn out. It's when we forget how much we once wanted to care. It's when we forget how important it is to us personally to effectively make a difference for others, to ease their pain and suffering, to make it better somehow. If we can't do this for others, then what's the point? Our desire to care in and of itself is not enough to bring us the bedside experiences we crave. We must find a way to act on our initial pure desire to care in order to create our own professional and personal satisfaction.

I thought I had been caring all along. But now I get it. Thinking we are caring does not make us caring. Wanting to care does not mean we care. It is our connection to others that allows us to feel love, joy, bliss, happiness, and what we're all searching for in our work: satisfaction. Real, authentic connection to patients is what it is all about. The ability to feel connected, to feel cared for, to feel that you yourself care, to feel you matter and make a difference, is what gives meaning and significance to our lives and purpose to our work. Yet for years "they" have been telling us to keep our distance. *Stay clinical, don't get attached, don't lose your objectivity. You won't be able to handle it!*

As I looked back over my life and my clinical career, searching for the missing ingredient, I saw it all in a new light. I saw how, when I'd finished my residency and begun my AIDS practice, I had no medicines, nothing to give my patients—so what I gave them was me, my concern, my interest and advice. I got to know them, who the people in their lives were and how they lived. I touched them. I did hands-on healing with them. If they missed an appointment, I called them to see how they were. I held them when they were overwhelmed or in tears. I went to see them in the hospital when they overdosed on the pills I'd prescribed for their nerves or their pain. I went to their funerals. And I remembered how engaged I was with that work, how happy I was. When I had no medicine to give except my care and concern, I saw how powerful that energetic medicine actually was, not only for me, but for my patients as well. There was not even one patient who ever complained.

I remembered the rural Tennessee hospitals where I'd worked in the '80s, where we had blue pills for their nerves, red pills for their headaches, green pills for their stomach pains and white pills for their colds. Yeah, they were placebos, but I administered them myself and I sat at the patients' bedsides afterward, because the lab tech and the X-ray tech were only "on call" and we did not call them in unless the patients were dying. If they needed a shot, we gave them a shot of salt water or saline. We had almost nothing to give except our presence, our connection, and our care. And I remembered how they felt better, how they said thank you, how they came back and asked for more of those blue pills.

I remembered the day in my urologist's office when he told me that he was going to have to amputate my only remaining, though diseased and cancerous, testicle, which I desperately wanted to hold on to. I remembered how devastated I was when he told me that they did not make fake testicles anymore, because of the silicone breast implant debacle, and how this was the straw that broke the camel's back. I fell apart and sobbed bitter tears for what seemed like an eternity. I remembered how he wrapped his arms around me and held me until the tears stopped. How he looked me in the eye and said, this is awful, this is hard, this is horrible, but I want you to know that I am going to do everything I can to get you through this, and you will be healthy and whole again, I promise. I felt his care. What my urologist did for me is not tangible, it is not a core measure, and he couldn't even bill my insurance company for it. But even then I knew that his care, his connection, his concern, initiated my healing.

In all these cases, I was touched or I touched another—not physically, but energetically, with the human heart. This is clearly not something tangible, but something even more powerful than tangible things. And this was what I could have done, what I did not do, to make things better for the giant man with the purple cow affliction and for myself as well, to ease our shared suffering. I could have got present, connected with him and empathized with him, treated him with human dignity. It was finally clear to me that in order to be fully engaged, happy and satisfied with the work I was doing, I would have needed to clear the distractions, the worries and concern for me, so that I could clearly care for him.

As soon as this missing piece of the puzzle became clear to me, I promised myself that from this moment on I would be different, just as I had promised myself (even though ten years had passed) that I would live a different life if God would spare my life and let me survive cancer a second time. I had vowed then that I would connect to the "more in life." What I now realized was that there is more to the "more" to life—more to care—than what is physical, tangible and measurable, more than what we can see. I vowed I would never forget that **everything that is good and sweet in this world belongs to the unseen realm, and the only way to tap into it and enjoy it is through our connection to someone else**.

What Care Isn't

I believe that inside the clinical encounter it is possible for us to "do" all the right things, cross all our t's and dot all our i's, and still completely omit the intangible ingredient our patients are expecting—care. This "disconnect" is what leaves us and our patients feeling flat and empty at the end of the encounter. Yes, we ask questions. We determine what the problem is and we take steps to fix it. We do our clinical exam. We order tests. We interpret the results. We give medicines. We write prescriptions, generate very detailed discharge instructions full of legal disclaimers and tell them what to do next and where to follow up. But if we maintain our professional distance, when we walk out of the exam room, the patient is often bewildered or confused, asking, "Is that it?" We often seem taken aback or surprised in turn as we respond: "Yes, you can go now."

Then we are the ones to be bewildered or confused when they wonder, to our amazement, "You mean you're not going to admit me?" We must be going to admit them, they think, because they feel we haven't "done anything." "What do you mean, we haven't done anything? You were triaged, we made a chart, you had a history and physical exam, you had blood tests, urine tests, X-rays, an EKG, a CAT scan and IV, medicines to make you feel better—what do you mean, we did not do anything? We did all sorts of 'things'!" Herein lies our frustration on both sides of the stethoscope. What our patient is really saying is, **where is the care I came for**? And what we are saying is that we gave it to you—our healthcare is the diagnosis, the care plan and the medicines. It is the X-ray, the splint, the pain medicine, the crutch and the phone number to make the follow-up appointment with the specialist. But these "physical things," these goods and services are not the intangible and unique ingredient known as care that the patient came for.

So what is this stuff, this intangible "thing" called "care," that our patients are looking for, this "stuff" that we are not giving to them? We work in a hospital and we work in the area of emergency care, but there is intensive care, critical care, surgical care, hospice care, end-of-life care, prepartum care and care for the newborn.

We are all familiar with childcare, day care and the increasingly popular adult day care. We have in-home care and extended-care facilities. Everyone is interested in quality of care, and we ask our patients if they are satisfied with our care.

None of us like to deal with car care, but some of us are just plain crazy about lawn care, and what would we do without doggy day care? We spend fortunes on skin and hair care. And how many times were we disappointed early in life when our parents refused our requests for more toys because "you don't take care of the ones you've already got"?

We use the word *care* so frequently and attach it to so many things that it seems familiar, even ordinary. We say we "care" about the people in Haiti and the unemployed and homeless here at home. When we are not interested in something we say we don't care. When we make a mistake people say we are careless. When our hearts get broken we act like we could care less.

No matter how you slice it or how you dice it, our care always involves our attention or focus. We care about our parents' safety or our children's happiness. We care for infants, the disabled, the sick, the injured and those who are not capable of caring for themselves. To care **for** someone moves our attention beyond the place it rests when we care **about** them, and it seems to imply some sort of sense of responsibility for the well-being or safety of the other—like when we care for our patients. Caring about someone or something is passive and does not really accomplish anything. Caring for someone is an active process, and participating in this process can change everything for us, as well as our patient.

When we care for someone with a problem, our natural human tendency is to want to solve the problem. When we see suffering, we want to see it end. If someone is hungry, we give them food. If someone is homeless, we find them shelter. If someone has a headache, we give them Tylenol. These "cures" are all ways in which we express our "care," but we must be ever so careful not to mistake these acts for care itself. Care is something much more organic, more primal, even more spiritual. Cure exists in the physical world, while care exists in the world of thoughts and emotions—those of the giver and those of the receiver. **Cure and care are worlds apart**.

If I have said it once, I have said it a thousand times to the doctors and nurses I work with. Patients don't come for the X-ray, the lab tests, the diagnostic interpretations, the medicines or the paperwork. They come because they have a problem that they can't fix, and they want someone to "care" about it. They come because they want someone with more knowledge, more understanding, more resources, more power, to care enough about what is going on for them, to understand what they are going through and to grasp what they are up against. They want someone who has the capacity, the knowledge, the wisdom and the expertise to comprehend the entirety of their situation, not just their disease or injury; someone who can empathize with them, and then offer advice or treatments from there.

Let's face it, anybody can get sick or be injured, and illness or injury can effectively take everything away from you. Rich, poor, educated, uneducated, no matter who you are, your life as you know it, your family, your finances, your resources, your sense of security and safety, can all be consumed. When you are the patient with a problem, you have no control. It doesn't matter if you are Gilligan, Thurston Howell, the Skipper, the Professor, Mary Ann or Ginger, you can still end up on a desert island.

When disease or illness threatens your life, you may find yourself suddenly terrified, scared to death, overrun with questions you have no answers to. Your whole understanding of the cosmos and your place in it, your spirituality, your religion, your friendships and family relationships all come into question. In this place of overwhelm, you may not be capable of exercising any meaningful or sound judgment—and **worse yet, you know it. Suddenly you are helpless, and often hopeless. It is from this place that you go to the hospital for care.** And in this place, providing the diagnosis is not care. Knowing the best treatment plan is not care.

When I was sick with cancer and it had become clear to my urologist that the disease had metastasized, he sent the oncologist to see me while I was still in the hospital, recovering from the surgery. The oncologist told me in the morning that I needed to start chemotherapy the very next day. Later in the afternoon, he came back and said, "We need more tests. I have to send you for an MRI and I can't get you in until next week." Wait—you said my life depended on starting tomorrow, now you want me to wait a week? He said, "Yes, that is what I am telling you, you have to wait a week and you need to get an MRI first." In that moment, did I feel I was receiving care? No! I was angry, I was frightened, and I did not feel he cared at all—unlike my surgeon, who reassured me that he would do whatever it took to get me through this. Rationally, I knew that the oncologist must care; I just could not feel his care.

Entering into the Pain

Before we can make caring for others our primary concern, we need to really understand what *care* means. I looked to our literature for help; there was little there. I looked to psychology and psychiatry, but saw only that the "therapeutic relationship" is necessary—not well characterized or defined. There was nothing that would tell us exactly how to create that sacred doctor-patient connection.

I looked to the nursing literature, the lay press, alternative medicine, philosophy, metaphysics, religion and spirituality. There was only one thing I read in all of my research into care that generated the epiphany I was searching for. It happened when I found Father Henri Nouwen, a Dutch-born Catholic priest who wrote roughly forty books, including *The Wounded Healer*, *The Life of the Beloved* and *The Way of the Heart*, just to name a few. He taught at the University of Notre Dame as well as Harvard and Yale, and he worked with people who suffered from developmental disabilities and/or mental handicaps. One of his most famous books, *Inner Voice of Love*, was written while he was struggling personally with serious clinical depression.

This learned and pious man thought about and wrote volumes on the topic of care. He knew that **our need for care—both to give it and to receive it—is rooted in the human condition itself**.

Please stop and take that sentence in. Humans are mortals; we all must face pain, suffering, disappointment, regrets and ultimately death. There are no exceptions. None of us are immune.

Father Henri teaches us that the word *care* comes from the Gothic *kara*, meaning "to lament, to grieve, to experience sorrow, or to cry out with." He says, **"The friend who can be silent with us in a moment of despair or confusion, who can stay with us in an hour of grief and bereavement, who can tolerate not knowing . . . not healing, not curing . . . that is a friend who cares."**

Our own dictionary describes care as a state of mind in which one is troubled, worried, anxious or concerned. No wonder we in a clinical setting have developed some confusion around the concept of care. Father Henri tells us the truth of the matter is that **all of us, without exception, "are uncomfortable with an invitation to enter into someone's pain before doing something about it." But the essence of care doesn't lie in doing something about the pain—it lies in entering into it, freely and wholeheartedly.**

When I was volunteering at the free clinic, with HIV-positive patients, when I had no medicines to give them and I learned how to give of my self to them, I believed that I helped them manage the stressors the disease brought, that I was offering them good advice, that I was providing them with comfort and reassurance. Then the one person who loved me, the one person who meant the most to me, was diagnosed with HIV. The news shattered our entire life. What if he had given it to me? How would we be able to make love? How long would he live? What would we do with the time he had left? There was nothing I could do to fix it for him. Just as with the patients I had been caring for, there were no pills or treatments to cure him. That diagnosis, however, somehow brought me to care for him more than ever, in ways that I never dreamed were possible—ways that I never thought I was capable of caring.

When my father had the best surgeons, in the best facility, for the best five-vessel heart bypass surgery available anywhere, but had a huge stroke while on the operating table, everything suddenly changed, for him, for my mother, for me, my brother, my sister-in law and their three children. When the neurosurgery fellow showed me my dad's CAT scan and I saw the images for myself, I audibly gasped. Half of his brain was gone! The look he shot me said clearly that he understood how devastating this was. There was nothing to be done, and yet somehow that knowing glance made everything better for me; it made it possible for me to think clearly enough to deliver the news to my dad and to support my mom through the process.

My mom showed me, through the next eight years that Dad was an invalid, what care, empathy and compassion are really about. When she was diagnosed with terminal esophageal cancer, even though I was a doctor, I was powerless to change things for her. I cared for her just the same. And in the eighteen days that followed her diagnosis, until the moment she took her last breath, she managed to care for me, my brother and his wife, and her grandchildren too. My mom never stopped caring. On the day she passed away, it was almost as if she had said, *Pay attention, son, I am about to show you how to lay your body down with grace, style and dignity. I have one last lesson to teach you.*

The immutable truth is that when the unthinkable happens, we all depend and count on the expert and compassionate understanding and advice of our doctors and hospitals. We all want our doctor to care about "us." We want our doctor to have our best interests at heart, even if he has another patient or he is asleep and it is 2 a.m. What this means is that **in our providers of medical care we want to find someone who can fully comprehend our awful situation, but even more importantly, someone who has the capacity for *kara*: to stay in the awful place and share our pain, feel our pain, validate our pain, understand our loss and lament with us**.

Traditionally, we are told not to connect with our patients, to stay professional, keep our distance. Our fear is that if we really care, their grief—our grief—will overwhelm us. How often do people tell you that they could never do what you do, that they don't know how you do it? It's high time we dismantled that simple untruth. It won't kill us. We are not going to die. It is only when we connect, when we feel the pain of another, when we share a moment of our shared humanity together, that we actually become fully alive Make no mistake about it, it is when we avoid that connection that we lose our power to make a difference, and this renders us powerless. This makes us victims. This is the reason we suffer from a victim's disease, the secondary PTSD of compassion fatigue and professional burnout.

It is only in those moments at work when we do become fully alive in this way that we can heal the effects of compassion fatigue and burnout within ourselves. Our shared experiences with our patients and their families of this nature are more powerful than any drug or surgery we can deliver as cure. The healing power of these shared experiences extends to both sides of the stethoscope.

Hard-Wired to Care

I have already shown you that we in medicine are afraid of this empathetic connection, as we have bought into the myth that we can't get close to patients—that empathy will make us suffer, and that we will lose our objectivity and make bad decisions. That is just not true. What is true is that we can't tolerate the pain without wanting to do something about it. This is why we have become so fascinated with technology, with the science of medicine—with the cure. We have mistakenly believed that if we could just fix it, we would not have to enter into their pain. But nothing could be further from the truth. For our healing to be effective, we *must* be willing to step into the pain of the one we would hope to heal. We must be willing to exercise our own capacity for *kara*. When we do this, then it *is* as if we take a piece of their pain away from them as they sense in some unseen, intangible way that we know exactly how they feel.

I'll say it again: our patients did not come for the X-ray, the splint, the crutches, the note for work, the antibiotic, the CBC or the EKG. They came to us because they wanted someone to care. Our confusion blurs the distinction between care and the expression of care. Our care generates the action that delivers the tissue to dry the tear or the bandage to stop the bleeding. But the action isn't all that matters, and often it's not even the first thing that matters.

Sometimes the tears need to flow and the blood needs to drip just a little to get the patient to the place where healing can begin.

It's healing not just for our patients, but for us. Let's look at some eloquent and exciting neuroscience from researchers Matthieu Ricard and Tania Singer. They show us, using the MRI scanner, that when we empathize with a person who's suffering, the area of our brain that registers suffering is activated in the same way and at the same location as the brain of the person we are empathizing with. This is the state we're in when we're faced with a suffering patient and we're feeling bad, feeling sad, thinking how awful it is for him or her. This state is what I call "stand-alone empathy," and if we stay in it, we suffer too.

But when we move from lamenting how bad things are to actively **wanting things to be better**, we're shifting from empathy into compassion—and when we bring the component of compassion into our experience, it's like the floodgates open. According to Ricard, every atom of suffering becomes soaked with loving kindness and the experience—physical and emotional—transforms into something much different. The change shows up in our brain too: when compassion is activated, all the areas in the prefrontal cortex and limbic system that handle distress, fear and pain are deactivated and the dopamine-rich wholesome centers, the ones that generate positive emotional states, kick in.

This is why the belief in keeping our "professional distance" is flawed: it looks at empathy as an isolated event instead of seeing its role in the process of connection. We'll come back to Ricard and Singer and look more closely at this neurochemical change later on in the book. For now, what I want you to understand is that, in a sense, "compassion fatigue" is a misnomer, because while stand-alone empathy can hurt—and lead to burnout simply because we get stuck in it. No one has ever taught us how to move beyond the angst and sadness of empathy—it's activating our compassion, our desire to care, that moves us past the pain. I believe that compassion cannot fatigue, it can only enlarge, engage and empower the one who feels compassion for another. The real name for compassion fatigue should be "Empathetic Overload."

As a society we have become preoccupied with speed. We live in a world where we have come to expect instant answers, instant solutions and even instant cures. In medicine we have advanced, technologically speaking, in powerful and amazing ways. We have the technology today to do what would have been considered miraculous just a few years ago. But as we focus on the technology, we blur the distinction between care and the expression of care (that is, the cure) even more. Cure without care involves us only with rapid diagnosis and treatment; rarely does it solve the underlying problem, and in the meantime it completely moves us away from the human experience of care.

In order for patients to feel our care, we must be willing to satisfy **our own need to answer the cry of someone who is hurting**. We must reconnect with our original, primal desire to help. The real purpose of care is not to fix anything, but rather to acknowledge the depth and reality of the human experience. When we mature as caregivers, we will see that our compassionate care is born from our own feelings and fears, born from our understanding that we are all merely mortals and in truth dependent on each other for solace. Our ability to truly care comes from knowing that when our time comes, someone will be there to lament and grieve with us. None of us wants to "go it" alone!

I believe that humans are hard-wired to care. Our desire to care for others is what led us into our professional roles in the first place. But there are so many things distracting us from the business of caring that our patients do not feel our care, even though they get the cure.

This is especially true when the problem or the condition is "minor." We all know that the very sick ones are easy to care for: they are always appreciative and they almost always, if they have the capacity to do so, say thank you. *If only we could just take care of sick people . . .* How many times have you heard that one? What happens when we care for patients who aren't so ill, the patients with bumps, bruises, colds, headaches and other minor conditions? For the sake of simplicity, let's just take a quick peek at those humans we care for after a minor trauma.

How many adults do we see in our departments who have had some sort of blunt trauma to an extremity? How many of them go home with a negative X-ray? How many of them get an ice pack and some pain medicine, or an Ace wrap, while they are in our departments? What about the patients we see who've hit their heads? How many of these have a negative CAT scan and get an ice pack, pain medicine and possibly some stitches before they go home? How many of these sorts of "minor" patients do we see in our departments all across America? Thousands? Millions? And how many of these patients answer the questions on the Press-Ganey Survey—"The staff cared about me as a person" or "The doctor took time to listen"—with Fair, Poor or Very Poor?

My guess is that most of them do. Because they could tell that we felt we had other, sicker patients to tend to. They felt our distraction. They never got our attention. We never had the chance to tell them we were sorry that this happened to them. Truth be told, we may have been on the way to their room to give them the good news that the X-rays were normal when we got pulled into the critical room to resuscitate a patient.

When our patients with the bumps or the bruises were young children and something similar happened, they probably went running to their moms. Dr. Mom picked them up, assessed the damage, reassured them, told them it would be okay, sealed the deal with a kiss and they were on their way. Many of them remember these encounters fondly. If there was a Press-Ganey survey about Dr. Mom, I am certain she would get Good's and Very Good's. Think of this as the perfect emergency encounter.

Why? Because Mom's main focus was to care. She made an intimate connection with them; she paid attention to what was going on. As a matter of fact, she gave them her undivided, full attention, and she felt their pain as if it were her own— she would gladly have taken the physical pain upon herself rather than see her child hurt. She lamented with them and the pain was gone almost as quickly as it came. No X-ray. No Ace wrap. No Tylenol. Just a little old-fashioned kindness and compassion. None of this cost even a dime, and it took hardly any time.

If I could share only one concept with all of modern medicine, it would be this: **Don't confuse care with the expression of care, the cure, the fix or the solution. They are not the same.** Our patients do not come to us only for a cure, so *delivering* only the cure is unsatisfying to both our patients and ourselves. Yes, our patients are hoping beyond all hope that there is a cure and that we can deliver it, no matter what the hour or what the cost. **But be clear: the ability to care has nothing to do with a cure. They are two separate things entirely.**

Making the Connection

I now know that I am only cheating myself when I stay "professional" or "clinical," when I don't take advantage of the opportunity to connect energetically with my patient. You see, deep down, I believe we all know that everything that we are looking for in the clinical encounter, and everything our patients need, exists here, in this unseen, immeasurable connection, and we in modern medicine can no longer ignore its existence. True care only exists in this unseen place of quantum energies—this place where the seen and the unseen are intimately intertwined, where the energies of life itself are found—and the only way to enjoy it is to jump in, get present and get connected. The only way to recover from burnout and compassion fatigue, the only way we can restore our own humanity, recover from our own emotional wounds, is to jump into an emotional connection with our patients. Our experience of generating compassion for them while in connection with them will change the neurochemistry in our own brains, and as a result, both will feel better.

None of us can go home at the end of the shift and feel satisfied with "I did my job the way I was supposed to. I stayed clinical. I stayed objective. I did not get involved with my patients and their drama. I charted well. I billed well and I was professional and efficient. I crossed my t's. I dotted my i's." This satisfies no one. Our collective dissatisfaction comes from the fact that we omit the intangible piece of care, the true care, the compassion, the fact that there is a hurting human in front of us, looking for us to care for them.

I now know that dissatisfaction is never the problem. Dissatisfaction, frustration, fear, resentment, pain, anger and guilt are all results of the problem. This is why our efforts to increase satisfaction fail. Once we can agree on the problem, the solution will become obvious, for in the problem the solution already exists. Through my failures, through my illnesses, through my experiences, I believe that I have clearly identified the problem.

The problem is that the intangibles, the authentic connection, the concern, the empathy, the unseen, the immeasurable, are an essential component of the healing equation on both sides of the stethoscope—yet these intangibles have no place in the clinical encounter as we know it. This is why we're frustrated—both givers and receivers of care—and some of us are so frustrated that we are angry.

The solution, the only way we can go home at night after we have done our job, is to know that we have been present, that we have been connected, that we have done everything, given our all, given true care. Only then we will feel that we earned our satisfaction, made a difference and changed things in a meaningful way for our patients and ourselves. Only then we will have had a good day.

As we go forward together on our journey, I will show you how to identify the source of your dissatisfaction for yourself and give you tools, techniques and perspectives that will allow you to fix the problem and generate immeasurable amounts of satisfaction for yourself, your patients and all those you work with or encounter in a work day. I will teach you exactly what I've learned: that to care for someone else, I have to get *me* (my baggage, my ego, my defenses and my preconceived notions) out of the way and make it about *them*, the patient, the family, the nurses, the other attending physicians. I have to bring the intangibles into the equation. I have to make the connection.

In looking for a way to get present and connected with my patients, I have realized two very important things. I disconnect when I am worried about what is going to happen to me in the future, so I need to find a way to let go of my fears about the future. And I've realized that I fear the future when my focus is on me, when I am worried about what will happen to me, what will become of me. What I learned is that when my focus shifts to you, the patient, or whoever happens to be in front of me at the moment, I can instantly let that go. Instantly I am present. When I sincerely ask the question *How can I help you?* and truly listen for the answer, I am instantly connected.

I have come to understand that my professors were not lying when they taught me in medical school that medicine is both and art and a science. The problem is that we, in Western medicine, only pay attention to the science, to the physical, the measurable and the objective. They never taught me the *art* of medicine in medical school or residency.

This art of medicine, how to work with the unseen and the intangible, is what I will teach you here. I have given language and vocabulary to that which we cannot measure or quantify. I have developed tools that will allow you to work with the quantum energies involved in the simple and basic action of human care.

Bringing these two worlds together, the seen and the unseen, the art and the science, is the only solution to our problem of dissatisfaction in healthcare today. This is where the magic and miracles in medicine can happen.

These days, I am excited to go to work. I love my job and I love the people I work with. Paying attention to the "more" to life, the important things, the unseen, the intangible, is what lets me feel great, happy, energized and successful at the beginning, the middle and the end of each shift. For me, this is what the practice of medicine or nursing, this is what being a healthcare provider or caregiver, is all about.

My passion is to share my tools, perspectives and insights so that you too can get out of your own way, get present, get connected and give true care so that you can feel complete and whole once again. So that you can transform from healthcare worker to healthcare hero and experience again the joy and fulfillment you so badly wanted to create when you decided that this was the career for you. I promise you that once you are armed with these tools and techniques, you will feel the way I do. Better then ever, the best ever!

None of us can leave our souls or our emotions at the entrance to our jobs every day and expect to feel whole and complete. My pain, my suffering, my despair and that crazy big guy with the flying purple cow problem taught me that I could do more, I could be more and I could have real and lasting satisfaction. All of this I have learned and applied to my life has brought me back to life, real life. I am no longer suffering from compassion fatigue or empathetic overload. I am no longer suffering from the secondary PTSD of professional burnout. I have won my humanity back. I am now really living a life that is meaningful, filled with purpose, significance, meaning, passion and excitement. And I am not stopping until I bring satisfaction and fulfillment back home to you: today's doctors, nurses, patients and hospitals. We have all done without it for far too long.

Since that epiphany, that aha moment, nothing in the Emergency Department has changed, except for me—and those who have watched me, learned from me and done the same for themselves. This is what I want you to have as well. You can change your life as well as the lives of those you care for. It is not easy, and it does take commitment and hard work. But at the end of the day, there is nothing better than knowing that you gave your all, you cared, you made a difference and you changed the world, one patient at a time.

Chapter 4

Quantum Satisfaction

When I beat cancer and I got another chance at life, I realized that there was more to it than I'd been living. There was more than the car, the house, the partner, the job, the title and the degree, there was more than the physical things in this life, and I wanted more. I felt that if I were to die then, my life would have been a tragedy. I had not yet had a chance to leave my mark.

I have already told you that I want it all. I wanted—and I still want—to know, at the end of the day, that my time on this planet meant something. I still want the best physical things this world has to offer, but I also want to know that I was connected to others, that I was significant in the big scheme of things. I want to know that I left my mark, that I made things better for others. I want to know that my life had value. Today and every day, in real time, I want to know deep in every fiber of my being that what I do is meaningful. I want to know that because of who I am and what I do, I am making the world a better place.

Each and every day, I want to know that I am powerful, that I am accomplished, that I am a master at my craft. I want the internal "feel good" that happens when I use all of my talents, all of my knowledge, all of my wisdom to care for a patient. I want to know that my care makes a difference for them and nurtures me at the same time.

This feeling of mutual satisfaction, this lasting, timeless fulfillment, is the "more" that I want from life and from my practice of medicine—the more we all want. I crave it, I need it and I am willing to do whatever I have to do to get it. I suspect that you want it just as badly as I do.

I am going to tell you a story about one of those times when I got "more" from life, a time in my clinical career when I got what I have wanted from the time I was two years old and bandaging those stray dogs in my parents' backyard. This one case provided me with what I wanted when I took the MCATs and applied to medical school. What I wanted when I was chief resident. What I wanted when I sat for board certification. What I still want. What I will probably always want. This one case makes everything I have been through in my life worth it. If I never did another thing in medicine, I would know, because of this case, that I'd made a difference.

Inside the Emergency

Step back in time with me for a little while. I had just returned to work after beating my cancer and getting my second chance at life. I wanted "more" now more than ever. I had just started a great new job in a busy ED with lots of trauma and a large pediatric population. This was the first nationally accredited chest pain center in the country, and I felt very lucky to have landed a clinical position here. I was full of enthusiasm and optimism.

It was in my first weeks of working in this particular emergency department and we were still in the "getting to know you" period. None of the staff had seen me work clinically, and they were still unsure of my skills. Could I cut the clinical mustard? Would they feel confident bringing the sickest of the sick to me? Would I know what to do? Truth be told, I had not worked in a long time, and I was in the same boat. I was a little nervous, wondering if my skills had gotten rusty while I was out of the game.

It was early on my shift on a weeknight and I was working with an older, more experienced, really talented emergency physician. The emergency department was busy as usual, and his beds were all full as it was near the end of his shift. I would be working the overnight. Suddenly the squad radio went off. The medics were traveling hot—lights and sirens—with a four-year-old boy in cardiac arrest from a house fire. CPR was in progress. There was no IV. There was no airway. There was no way for the medics to give any medications without these. The boy was in asystole—the monitor showed a flat line.

For a moment, after that radio call, you could hear a pin drop. A hush and seriousness descended upon the entire department. You could sense the call to action. This was no ordinary case, and we were all aware that we could no longer be just ordinary people. Without a word, everyone, including me, knew and automatically assumed their positions on the team. Since they did not know my clinical skills yet, they wanted the more senior doctor to take this case. Disappointed, but relieved at the same time, I watched as the nurses made one of the other doctor's beds available so they could give this boy the best.

I stood by as the medics and the child, lifeless on the stretcher, rolled past my desk. The mother and father, crying, followed close behind. You could smell the smoke on the firemen. The energy all around was intense, surreal. I knew it would be my job to take care of the rest of the department and triage while they worked on the boy.

It was not very long, though, before one of the nurses came to me with a look of despair on her face and took me by the hand. Her look simply said *We need your help* as she silently led me past his frantic parents, through the curtain, into the bedside space. I can still remember it as if it were happening right now. Laying all consequences aside, this heroic nurse had taken me from the sidelines and "into the emergency." I was now in the place that I lived for, the place I had spent my whole life training to be.

Laying there on the stretcher was the flawless body of the four-year-old boy. The doctor had sweat on his forehead and a tear on his cheek. He and the nurses, struggling to obtain IV access for the medications, were all choked up—they all had children of their own. The respiratory therapist was bagging the patient, while the medic, dripping with sweat, was doing the chest compressions. Whenever he stopped, the ominous flat line on the monitor revealed just how lifeless this innocent four-year-old body was.

The physician filled me in on what had happened. Listening to the story, I understood that this boy was a mischievous little four-year-old and I instantly identified with him. What had happened was that while the rest of his family was watching a movie downstairs and eating popcorn, he had slipped away and was playing in the bedroom upstairs. He'd stuck something in a wall socket that caused a spark, blowing the lights out, and a fire had erupted. He must have realized something bad had happened and become frightened—maybe worried he would be blamed and punished—because he hid under his bed.

Flames soon engulfed the floor below and the family fled outside to safety. In the confusion, it took a few moments to realize Adam was missing. By this time the house was an inferno and smoke had filled the second floor. His father rushed back desperately to find him. Soon he was cut and bleeding from breaking windows to gain access to the upstairs, but his son was nowhere to be found.

The firemen pulled him out of the house for his safety, promising to find his son for him. Dad, mom, and all Adam's brothers and sisters stood in the cold night air as they watched their home being destroyed, begging and praying to see their brother pulled out alive. When a fireman finally emerged from the flames with Adam in his arms, it did not take long for them to realize that things were very bad.

As the senior physician shared this story, I moved closer to the bedside and asked his permission to get involved. There was not a mark on the little body before us. No scrapes. No cuts. No burns. No soot. As he'd lain underneath that bed hiding from his parents, Adam had been overcome with smoke and carbon monoxide. Even though his body looked so perfect and pink, the monitor continued to show a flat line.

To everyone's relief, I was able to get the IV started. As I moved to the head of the bed to secure the airway and place the ET tube, the nurses secured the IV and started fluids. The doctor began to give the medicines. Both optimism, that we could save this boy, and terror, that he might not survive intact, filled the room. We all feared that this boy could be brain-dead.

I recognized that I was in the zone, that place where it is as if I can step outside my ordinary self, observe myself, and see, hear and feel everything going on around me. I could hear Adam's parents outside the curtain. I could sense the concern of the medics and the firemen, also standing just outside. I could hear, between the sobs and tears, the clinical conversation between the nurses and the doctor.

As I checked my equipment and got ready to pass the tube, I heard a voice inside my head say, "Look, you are not God. You just do what you do. You give this boy everything you can to see if you can get him that second chance at life. You do for him what your doctors have done for you."

I placed the ET tube on the first pass. Respiratory therapy quickly got him on the ventilator and the medicines began to take effect. Then, as if by magic, his heartbeat spontaneously returned. CPR was discontinued and soon he had a blood pressure.

Finally, we could all exhale. Everyone's relief was palpable. Everyone then looked to me to see what was next. I handed control of the case back to the original doctor and stepped out to give his parents the update. I spoke optimistically, being cautious about prognosis, but also careful to feed their hope and prayer that Adam would be OK.

Then I took Dad into an exam room and got the nurses to formally make him a patient so that we could tend to his own injuries. Mom was overwhelmed, so I helped her get in the mindset that would help her to be strong and be ready to make decisions on her son's behalf, reminding her that her love for him would give her all the strength and courage she needed. She could break down later, but right now, she had to rise to the occasion.

Still inside the emergency, as the helicopter took off transporting Adam to the pediatric hospital, again I wondered, *What have we done? What if he never wakes up? What if he is a vegetable?*

What if? Again, that voice inside my head, told me, "Not your worry, you just do what you do, and do it the very best you can. That's your part."

Larger than Our Selves

Even though there was no way yet to know what the outcome would be, no way to know what would become of Adam, the truth is I had a great big smile inside me, possibly even on my face. I felt powerful. I felt a sense of accomplishment. If I wanted to know that what I did mattered, well, there was no doubt that what I had just participated in had just about all the meaning and significance you could ask for.

I knew what we all did had made a difference, and even though the outcome was still unknown, at least for the moment we had saved the day. But this was no time to stop at feeling satisfied. It was now the early hours of the morning. This was a forty-bed ED and all the rooms were full. More patients had come for care while we were all "inside the emergency," and triage was backed up. It was time to regroup and get back to the business of running the emergency department.

As the other physician, who'd been in charge when we were "inside the emergency," was turning his patients over to me and getting ready to go home, he thanked me. "You did a nice job," he said. It was a rare moment in any emergency department.

Before he left, he told me that he was remaining hopeful and upbeat about what the outcome might be. We talked about the fact that we can only do our very best and hope for the best. Everything else remains outside our control. He hugged me, another rare moment in the ED, and said good night.

I struggled through the rest of my shift, as did the nurses, the secretary, the medics and registration. We had just been on an emotional roller coaster and there was no time to process any of it. The only thing we could do was to band together to move through the massive amount of work that lay before us. There were colds, and coughs, migraine headaches, back pains, lacerations, suicidal patients, psychotic patients, intoxicated patients and chest pains. We also had grandmas who couldn't breathe and grandpas who couldn't pee even though their bladders were about to bust.

Patients were soon frustrated and angry again. They understood about the delays initially, but then they started saying, "Hey, that helicopter left hours ago. Where are my test results? I need more pain medicine. When are you going to discharge me, when will my room be ready, hey, what about me?"

IVs were started, splints applied, sutures placed, medications given, crutches dispensed, discharge instructions and prescriptions written. Rooms were cleaned and turned over, again and again. Ambulances came and went. Finally the shift was over. We'd made it. It was time to go home.

But you know what? Even though we'd worked really hard; even though we were told we did a good job, no, we were told we did a great job; even though some patients and their families were understanding, and others were upset and entitled; even though we were competent, efficient, prudent and caring, and had enjoyed performing at superhuman levels of functioning; I had to wonder, were we taking satisfaction home with us? The situation did not yet feel complete, because we were not certain that Adam was going to be OK. I spoke in the last chapter about making that vital connection with a patient. This night, I know I that I left still feeling connected to Adam and his family. I believe that we all remained connected, and I am certain that we all took "Adam" home with us that day.

Days passed, weeks passed, months even passed, and we regularly received updates from the nurses and doctors now caring for Adam. He was off life support. His lab work looked good. His chest X-ray was fine. Even his brain scan and EEG were fine. His eyes were open, yet he would not eat, he would not speak; he just lay there, staring off into space. Weeks passed and no improvement. He would not interact, not even with his mom. They had no choice but to place a feeding tube.

The time eventually came that Adam could no longer stay in the pediatric hospital. His insurance company said he was out of hospital days. Arrangements were made to send him to a pediatric rehab facility far away from his home. An ambulance took him north to his new home in rehab. Mom watched as they packed him into the back. Dad was at work, and the rest of her support system had stayed at home to care for the rest of her children. She followed behind the ambulance, alone.

Every day, since the moment the helicopter had taken Adam off to the pediatric hospital, I had prayed that he would improve, that his situation would get better. Every day I had wondered how his parents were coping. As we watched this process unfold during the months following the night of the fire, at least I felt some relief, that Adam was alive, that his tests were normal, but I still did not have the ultimate in satisfaction. I still worried what would be. Would he remain this way? What kind of a life would that be? Had I, had we, really given him a second chance at life, or had we actually diminished his chances for a happy life?

I thought we might never know, for once a patient goes to a rehabilitation facility, we rarely get any significant follow-up. Then one day in the emergency department I got that ultimate satisfaction experience. I had the pleasure of hearing the rest of Adam's story directly from his mom, who struggled, while she told the story, to contain a rambunctious, full-of-energy and mischievous-as-ever Adam by her side.

That day that she had followed behind the ambulance, after they arrived at the rehab facility and she'd walked into Adam's new room, she found the feeding tube was gone. Adam had pulled it out himself and he was in the middle of an animated conversation with his new nurse. After hugs, kisses and lots of tears, Mom asked Adam, "Why, why didn't you do this before?" He said, "I did not like those nurses and doctors at the children's hospital. They were mean."

Finally I felt the sweetness of victory. Satisfaction had arrived, not only for me, but for Mom, Dad, his brothers, his sisters, his aunts and uncles, his community, the doctor who was in charge inside the emergency that night, who'd wept silently as he attended to this child, the nurses who'd sobbed as they pushed the medicines and their co-workers hung the fluids, our hospital, the flight team and the pilot of the helicopter, the firemen, the paramedics, the pediatric trauma center, the rehab facility, for each and every individual who'd cared, who wanted to make a difference, who'd wanted to change things, to make things better. Finally it was clear that what we had done that night that fire destroyed Adam's house had made all the difference in the world.

What can we learn about satisfaction from this case, and what can we learn about its opposite from the case of the flying purple sex-crazed cows? In both cases, physically, I did very similar, if not the same, things. I assessed a situation, intubated a patient, gave life-sustaining meds. But there was a crucial difference. With Adam, I was fully present. I had no thoughts or concerns for myself. I did not keep my professional distance. I showed up, completely, in my entirety. I brought ALL OF ME, my mind, my intellect, my heart and even my soul, along with my initial pure and uncorrupted desire to care, to help, to make a difference. I brought it all to the bedside.

In Adam's case, I held nothing back. I connected completely. It was all about Adam, I empathized with his mom and dad, I was connected in empathy to the team I was working with—there was no room in my conscious awareness for me. I moved beyond that empathetic connection to a place of compassion, where I just wanted everything to be better for everybody involved. Everything that I said, all that I did, came from that place of compassion inside me. In the other case, my concerns were mostly for me, even though I didn't realize it at the time. I merely went through the motions while I was personally annoyed and distracted. You could say I had reason to be annoyed and distracted—the guy had tried to kill me, after all—but then you'd be missing an essential point about care.

In Adam's case, we were connected to our patient, each other and the family. None of us wore a plastic emotionless politically correct clinical face, and none of us had a smile on our face. None of us were thinking about ourselves, either. The firemen were not thinking about their own lives, their children or their wives, when they rushed into the flames to pull Adam out of that house. Somehow, all of our personal needs, including the need to use the bathroom, just dropped away. Adam's needs, his parents' needs, were, in the moment, all that counted. We were crying as we worked to save his life. We allowed ourselves to feel the anguish of the human condition then, and to lament with them—to feel their pain and take it on as our own. It was again our capacity for *kara* that allowed us this level of human experience, this level of shared connected compassion satisfaction.

Since Adam, I have had other, similar experiences, where all the necessary components come together in such a larger-than-life way, and I can think of no other type of experience in any part of my life where I am automatically and spontaneously more fully present and engaged with who I am, what I do and my desire to help.

As I think back on my career, I see that in every case where we "**step inside the emergency**" to battle death for our patients because they can't, we become larger than our ordinary selves, because the situation demands nothing less from us. This is why we want to be doctors, nurses, medics, firemen, techs, secretaries and even housekeepers in hospitals. We want to connect to that intangible energy, the energy of the hero. Did you ever notice, as in Adam's story, that when we are "**inside the emergency**," suddenly we act as a team—as one single unit? We become a hero working with a team of heroes. We don't bad-mouth each other or our patients. We automatically know where every piece of equipment we need is, even if we have not seen it or used it in years. We know which part of the body is our responsibility. We flawlessly anticipate each other's needs and fulfill them.

As I am passing the ET tube, the secretary is calling X-ray for the post-intubations film. The nursing supervisor mysteriously shows up and can suddenly nurse like she has been doing it forever, making the calls to get the helicopter here now, directing the secretary to get the tertiary care center on the line so our physician can speak to theirs. Registration is placing the family in the family room, getting them comfortable and coffee (a simple cup of coffee is transformed by kindness and compassion into something extraordinary) and helping them extract important numbers from their purse or the patient's cell phone. Security is way ahead of us, stepping up to control the crowd and the gawkers. We feel connected to each other. We feel connected to something larger than us.

There is no end to the feeling of satisfaction here, and it is circular, it lives on in perpetuity. This is the stuff that changes lives and changes (y)our world. Herein is where meaning, purpose, significance, power, accomplishment, happiness, fulfillment and joy live. This is the dream we all so desperately cling to—this is what all of us in healthcare really want, what we do the work for. And guess what, you can't see it, hear it, touch it, smell it or taste it. You can't bottle it and you can't sell it. It is not a tangible thing and it does not live in our world of physicality. It exists only in one place, inside the world of human thought and emotion. It lives in the "more to life." It lives only in our uniquely human consciousness.

The Quantum World

I hope that you have noticed, through the multiple places in this story where satisfaction shows up, that satisfaction feels good. You most probably like what you are feeling now, or what you were feeling when you got to the part of the story where Adam told his mom, that he did not like those nurses and doctors at the pediatric hospital because they were mean. How many times have you had to start an IV on a four-year-old when he was screaming bloody murder, shrieking at the top of his lungs, "No! Mommy! No!" How many times have you been perceived as mean, even though in reality you were being kind, compassionate and caring? This is how we know that our satisfaction lies in the giving itself: only we know for certain that we started the IV in the most compassionate and, to the best of our abilities, the most painless way possible, even if we don't get the thank you or the "wow, you are so amazing."

I would also like to point out to you that as you are reading this, wherever you might be—in your bed, your living room, at Starbucks, on the subway or even on the beach—it should be clear to you that satisfaction has nothing to do with your environment. Close your eyes for just a second and think about the most satisfying experience you ever had. Do you feel the satisfaction once again? Now open your eyes. What does that feeling of satisfaction have to do with the beach or the Starbucks? Absolutely nothing! To this day, I feel the satisfaction of Adam's story no matter where I am. I carry it with me always.

The sweetness of satisfaction exists only in one place. Real satisfaction only exists inside each and every one of us. Satisfaction does not exist in our environment. Satisfaction has nothing to do with our physical reality. Satisfaction also has nothing to do with time, as it exists beyond time. Satisfaction can't be perceived with our five human senses. None of us can see, hear, smell, taste or touch satisfaction.

Although we try, through patient satisfaction surveys and employee satisfaction questionnaires, we can't really measure satisfaction like we can measure speed, or temperature, or even quantify the force of gravity, but each of us recognizes satisfaction instantly "in" ourselves and "in" others.

We know when we have satisfaction. Somehow you sense that I am satisfied. Somehow I know when you are satisfied and when you are not. If it is not our five senses that we use to recognize satisfaction "in" ourselves and "in" others, what is it, then? Where does it exist? I believe that the key lies in that word, *in*: we recognize satisfaction *in* our hearts and minds, inside our personal world of thoughts and emotions, where, combined with our five-sense perceptual data, we create our personal consciousness. Consciousness is defined as the fact of awareness by our mind of our self in the world; consciousness emerges from the operations of our brain.

Einstein has taught us that everything is either energy or matter. If so, then our consciousness, which emerges from the operations of the brain (matter), must be energy. Consciousness is actually awareness of thoughts, which are not tangible, physical things; they are energy, and our consciousness of them is energy too. It is our consciousness that recognizes satisfaction in ourselves and others, and so satisfaction must exist in the same place consciousness does, in the world of energy—in Einstein's quantum world, named for the smallest unit of energy we can measure.

We use the energies contained in the quantum world every day in medicine. It does not bother us that we can't see X-rays, heat, ultrasound or microwaves. We don't care. We use them anyway. We use them because we have studied them and measured these unseen forces of energy. This is possible only because of advances in scientific progress, and because we now have the microscopes, the meters and the gauges that allow us to measure what we cannot measure with our five senses. We can't sense X-rays, and that is why those who work in X-ray wear badges that sense the S-rays for them, to protect them from too much exposure. But we use X-rays clinically hundreds of thousands of times each day.

With our thoughts and emotions, it's different. The reason that we in modern Western medicine ignore their power in our practice is because we can't yet scientifically measure and validate them. We do not yet have the technology to measure the energy of thought or emotion.

Yet none of us would deny their existence. They are a crucial component of the mystery of medicine, the art of medicine that we, in today's modern scientific age, have all but forgotten. It is time that we investigated the way our thoughts and emotions play a role in generating satisfaction for ourselves and for our patients, even if we have no way to measure them. We might even ask whether these might be the very source of healing—but that's a subject for another book.

X-rays, microwaves, infrared rays, thermal energy and light itself *can* be measured with today's instruments, and interestingly enough, as Einstein predicted, they all follow the same patterns and rules; they all behave the same. So working with these measurable energies becomes predictable. I believe that we can discern patterns in the workings of consciousness, too; we can look to quantum physics to help us understand the ways in which our thoughts and emotions work so that we can use them to our advantage and the advantage of our patients. They will become just another tool that we use to help others, except they won't generate something physical or tangible—they will generate the quantum energy of satisfaction.

Satisfaction on Both Sides of the Stethoscope

The profound satisfaction of caring for Adam came almost all on its own, spontaneously, because I and my co-workers were plunged "inside the emergency" by his situation—into that space where nothing matters but caring for the patient and connection is immediate and profound. What about those situations that don't put you in the zone—those ordinary interactions with patients, be they grumpy or grateful?

I promised you that, in this book, I would teach you how to create more and more really positive experiences at work where you help someone, they know you've helped them, and your care makes a difference for both of you. I promised you that I would show you how to use this knowledge to create more and more satisfaction for yourself at work by generating more and more positive experiences at work. You see, there is a way to systematically create the quantum energies of satisfaction. The process has seven steps, and you will go through these seven steps each and every time you want to create a really great experience for yourself and your patient. To help you fix the steps in your mind, I've chosen the mnemonic R.E.F.L.E.C.T.—especially apt because it also describes the process of looking inward for answers.

These are the steps:

1. **REMEMBER what you came here for.** Reconnect with your desire to care. Remember what you want from your work: the feeling good that comes from truly caring for others.

2. **EARN your satisfaction.** Realize you are responsible for your own satisfaction and that for it to last, you have to earn it.

3. **FORMULATE your plan**. Recalculate the transaction of care using the Perfect Equation.

4. **LOOK at your position within the transaction of care:** are you the cause or the effect? Reframe your position in the interaction with your patient.

5. **EVALUATE your results.** Recognize what you bring to the encounter. Is your giving care effective? If not, go to step six and begin again.

6. **CIRCLE BACK to the beginning.** Regroup when the encounter is over so you can do it all again. Remember your desire is to care. Look for a fresh opportunity to care again.

7. **TAKE CARE of yourself.** Restore and renew yourself by applying the quantum skills you've learned to energize and elevate every part of your life. Apply the tools of transformation so that you can transcend your present limitations.

At this point in our journey, we've already taken a couple of these steps together. If you've read this far, I hope you are ready to reconnect with the desire that brought you here—**to remember what you want and why you came to healthcare** in the first place. I hope it's coming back to you! You came here because you have a pure and simple desire to care, to help, to make things better for people.

This pure desire to help is hard-wired in you; it is part of who you are. And as Matthieu Ricard has shown us, when you actualize your desire to care while you're connected to your patient in the experience of compassion, all of the dopamine-rich feel-good centers in your prefrontal cortex light up. Neurologically, when we care, when we generate compassion for another while connected to them, we take advantage of our own human biological and neurological hard-wiring and this results in our feeling good. Humans are Hard-Wired to Care. It is the fact that we all bought into the myth that connecting to our patients is bad for us and bad for our patients, the fact that we don't routinely connect, that prevents us from feeling good as a result of our efforts to care.

Right now—and this is the reason I wrote this book, the reason you're still reading—you do not feel good often enough at work, in the place you came to realize your desire to help others. In step one, our goal is to always **Remember** why we came here, to this job, and what we want from it. We did not come here in the first place to start an IV, with or without an ultrasound machine, we did not come here because we wanted to do flawless five-level triage, we did not come here because we wanted to make a diagnosis or perform a history and physical exam. **We came here because we want to care and we want our care to make a difference**.

We came here because we want to be someone's hero. All heroes know that their personal satisfaction comes from only one place, from the act of saving the day for another. In other words, if we want satisfaction, if we want to feel good, we have to care for someone. We must always remember this: *We came here because deep down inside we want to care for someone in need.* And we know now that true care doesn't mean just giving a shot or setting a broken bone—it means connecting with our patients and letting them know we share their pain. To feel good at work, we have to step through our fear (and our training) and make an authentic connection with those we are caring for.

So, now that we know our job satisfaction comes through the act of caring for others (and now that we've investigated the distinction between care and cure), we will have to explore satisfaction to move on to step two. Again, if you're still with me, you may have reached this step on your own. It's where we realize where satisfaction comes from and how we access it—how we **Earn** it. To do this, we need to examine what we know about the nature of satisfaction.

Satisfaction always starts with a desire. You have to want something. Satisfaction is the realization of the desire, the actualized desire. Satisfaction is sometimes related to a physical object, but it is never the object itself. A classic example is the piece of paper your degree is printed on. The physical piece of paper represents the satisfaction you earned by achieving your dream or reaching your goal, but your satisfaction exists in your thoughts and feelings about that particular piece of paper, not in the paper itself.

My retelling of, and your reading of, Adam's story, showed us that satisfaction exists inside of us and that it has little, if anything, to do with our physical surroundings. Satisfaction is actually an internal state of being. Satisfaction is an identifiable, positive feeling, but it is not tangible. Satisfaction cannot be perceived with any of our five senses, but when we have satisfaction, we instantly recognize it, in our hearts or our minds, or perhaps both.

In Adam's case, we all got fully present. We put our own needs aside. We connected to Adam's parents and his situation. We wanted the best possible outcome. We used all of our training, experience, talents and skills. We (I) prayed for Adam. We (I) felt the almost unbearable, all-consuming, harsh pain of his parents, his brothers, his sisters and the community. We banded together and connected to each other. We became a team.

None of us judged Adam's parents for not covering the wall sockets with plastic plugs. None of us judged Adam's parents for not realizing that he was not with them watching the movie. We had empathy for his parents and we felt their pain. We found compassion for them. These are the things we do, the actions we take, in addition to performing the physical tasks of starting the IV and recording the vital signs, to earn our satisfaction whenever we step "inside the emergency." We feel accomplished when we earn our satisfaction by taking actions beyond the physical and include the human consciousness that contains our thoughts and feelings. In truth, satisfaction exists in only one place, the mysterious world of our personal consciousness.

No one can give you satisfaction. You have to create it for yourself. Think about the process of getting your degree. Did you work for your degree? Were you satisfied when you earned your diploma? **The *Jerry Maguire* "you complete me" fantasy never works. No one else will ever make you happy.** In relationship, you can find your own happiness and share it with another, but you can never make someone else happy. **No one can complete you**. Every therapy and every self-help book teaches us that you must complete yourself first in order to enter into a successful long-term partnership with another complete being. It is the same with satisfaction: in the end, we are all responsible for our own happiness, our own peace of mind, our own security—and we are all responsible for creating our own satisfaction for ourselves.

In order to have satisfaction, you have to work for it. It comes in an amount proportional to the effort you expend. Others can make us feel good or better, with a hug, by caring for us or lending a hand, but this feeling better is not true satisfaction. It's the one giving the hug or care or hand to you who feels satisfaction, because *you* feel *their* love and care.

So step two in our framework is **to realize that because of the very nature of satisfaction itself, you and I are responsible for creating our own satisfaction and we need to Earn it for ourselves.** We have to actively create what we want for ourselves. There is nothing passive about satisfaction. We need to take responsibility by coming to the understanding that we are the cause of our own satisfaction. This is the litmus test: if you do not have the satisfaction you want, then you are not doing what you need to be doing to earn it.

In Adam's case, I know that I cared. I know that the nurse who led me by the hand to the bedside cared. I know that the more senior physician cared. As a mater of fact, I know deep in my heart that everyone on the team that night cared. Being present, empathizing and feeling compassion that night were the keys to the formula that brought us all personal and job satisfaction; the key ingredients in the formula that we used to make ourselves feel good.

We've already explored the definition of care, looked at what care most definitely is *not* and seen what true care is. Care is not the same as cure; cure is tangible goods and services, and care is intangible, a phenomenon of energy. Now it's time to take the third step, where we look more closely at the *transaction* of care—the interchange we take part in every time we deal with a patient—and recalculate it according to a formula by which caring equals satisfaction every time.

Chapter 5

Formulating Our Plan of Care

Maybe now would be a good time for us to review what we have been discussing and see where we are on the journey to satisfaction:

1. So far, you've seen that step one on the journey is to **REMEMBER** what you want by reconnecting with your original pure and uncorrupted desire to care, and to remember where your satisfaction comes from: fulfilling your desire to care, to make a difference. You've seen the difference between care and cure: care is an energetic phenomenon, and cure is tangible goods and services

2. And you've taken step two. You know that you have to **EARN** your own satisfaction. You realize that you are responsible for creating your own satisfaction, your own feeling good, at work and in life. In order to feel good, you must give the energy of care while delivering the tangibles of cure.

3. Now you're ready for step three, where we'll **FORMULATE** your new plan by recalculating the "transaction of care" inside the patient encounter by using the Perfect Equation I'm about to introduce you to.

Defining True Care

Applying bandages, reading EKGs, starting IVs, pushing medicines, taking histories and the like for a living is sort of like making widgets for a living. People have been caring for other people successfully since the dawn of civilization, but the cures we have today have only become available recently, so care has nothing to do with the tangibles or technologies of "cure." While you trained and studied cure as a means to an end, to get the degree or the position that would allow you to care, in order to actually care you must focus on the intangible and work with your thoughts and emotions to create the quantum energies of satisfaction you crave. We will never feel satisfied if we only work with the physical widgets we use to provide cure.

So far, this is all pretty simple: reconnect to your uncorrupted desire to care—**remember what you want—then go for it**. Easy, right? Well, when it comes to the physical things you want, it is easy. Say you want a glass of water. You stand up, walk over to the sink, grab a glass and fill it with water. When you drink it, you have what you wanted. You have satisfaction. Getting the drink of water is like giving the "cure," the splint, the bandage, the crutch, the medicine, even the diagnosis and the treatment plan, straightforward and simple.

When you want a certain feeling, it's more complicated. For example, to feel loved. How easy is it to get love? This you can't do alone. This requires you to be in relationship with another. How easy is it to find true and lasting love?

In your job in healthcare, you are looking for a certain feeling that comes from your interaction with someone else, your patient. You have to be in relationship with your patients; your interaction is a process by which you give your thoughts and emotions to them, and this creates a change in their own thoughts and emotions, which results in a blend of both of your thoughts and emotions that feels good to both of you. It's a process I define as "True Care."

To care the way my colleagues and I cared for Adam "inside the emergency" means we get 100 percent present and focus our attention on the patient. No other patients can exist in our consciousness during this patient's "moment" of care. We have to connect to our patient. We must put his or her concerns, pain or suffering, no matter how severe or minor, in front of our own interests, even if it is just for a moment; we must let them know, see and feel that we acknowledge their pain as if it were our own, let them know that we are here with them and willing to walk alongside them through the pain, willing to share their burden for a minute or two, or even as long as it takes.

In the "emergency," this happens automatically—but we can make it happen under any conditions. Here is the process we can move through in the energetic world of human thought and emotion in order for our care to be effective and mutually satisfying. These are the six stages in the process for generating and delivering True Care:

1. **Presence:** Show up and get fully present. Look at the thoughts going on inside your head and put aside the ones that don't have to do with what's going on right now—those distracting thoughts of the work that's waiting for you or unfinished business at home. Now focus on the patient in front of you. Give him or her your full and undivided attention.

2. **Connection:** Connect with your patient. Introduce yourself and ask the patient's name. I often ask patients to tell me something about themselves that will help me remember who they are. Sometimes I shake their hand or touch their shoulder. I make eye contact as I ask what's going on with them, how are they feeling, where is their pain?

3. **Focus:** Make your patient's needs your focus. Put his fears, concerns and needs in front of your own. Show him some real human dignity. Remember, you are human too, and both of you deserve human dignity and human kindness.

4. **Empathy:** Start to imagine what this situation is like for her, what it would be like to walk in her shoes. Feel your patient's pain as if it were your own. Stay in this uncomfortable empathetic place with her until you feel things change—without offering to fix anything.

   Don't be afraid; this will not overwhelm you or drain you, because you're not going to stay here long. While you are here, think of it as the Sinatra moment. You know Frank always sang *Do-be-do-be-do*. Here you don't DO anything, you just BE with your patient. You will feel it when this empathetic connection is established. (You will feel it because the neurochemistry in your prefrontal cortex is changing, just as we saw in Matthieu Ricard and Tania Singer's MRI research. What you are feeling is real, and it's uncomfortable.

Then something happens on the other side of your stethoscope: your patient recognizes that you are feeling, at least to some extent, what he or she is feeling about the situation—that you understand the anguish or pain.

Next, something shifts in the quantum energies you are sharing. It shifts for you both, and you will sense it—or perhaps even hear or see it: a sigh, a sob, a relaxation of breathing, a softening of a fretful look, a slowing of the pulse.

5. **Compassion:** Now, you make the conscious decision to leave this painful place you share with your patient by turning on your own compassion. Feel your own desire for things to be better for them; for them to feel better, for the pain to lessen, their fear to dissipate, their anguish or their despair to soften. You do not yet speak or *do* anything. You just *be*. You are still only working with your thoughts and emotions, using your heart and mind.

This stage of the process will enlarge you, energize you and empower you. This is where the transaction of care occurs. This is where your mind affects matter, specifically the grey matter in your prefrontal cortex, and all the dopamine-rich feel-good life-enhancing centers light up like a Christmas tree on real-time MRI scanning, just as Ricard and Singer showed. You are in effect using your heart and mind to generate the Milk of Human Kindness (a special recipe of neurotransmitters) in your own brain, and this process, somehow, most probably through the scientific principle known as resonance, makes you and your patient both feel better.

This stage of the process is where you get to feel on a visceral level that you care, that what you do matters, that you make a difference and that you matter. This is the cure for your own compassion fatigue and (if compassion fatigue is left untreated too long) for your ultimate professional burnout.

6. **Action:** Finally, once you feel full of your own compassion, move on to the practical physical matters that will help make your patient's situation better or at least more tolerable.

That's it. Simple, really. Do not let this six-stage breakdown make you think that this is difficult or time-consuming. It is actually quite natural and can happen in only seconds—almost instantaneously, really, as one stage cascades after the next. The best part is that giving care this way not only changes everything for the patient, we benefit as well. To give care this way actually feels good. You don't feel drained and stressed. You feel empowered and so does your patient.

Stage four, the empathetic connection, is the defining stage for True Care, and the stage that diverges from all the medical training you've had. It's what makes the difference between customer service and real satisfaction—between the tools I am giving you and every other process you may have learned—because it asks you to get emotionally involved. Staying professional and detached, even if you say and do all the right things, just won't work. None of this is possible if your focus is on staying "clinical": warm and polite, but detached. Satisfaction only comes within reach for us when we get fully present, engaged with the thoughts and emotions of our patient in the quantum world.

Stage five, turning on your own compassion, is the "Holy Grail," the be-all and end-all solution for you to feel good (again) because you care. But make no mistake, it only works if you are willing and able to execute the first four stages. Can you, are you willing to, freely enter another's pain and suffering without first "fixing" it? When you are willing and choose to emotionally connect to the suffering before fixing it, you will have everything you ever wanted to feel as a result of your decision to become a care giver.

It's simple—but it's not always easy. If you are still reading this book, then I have to assume that you are having difficulty with this process because you don't feel so good at work, and you still want to know if and how you can feel good at work.

The Perfect Equation

Care is both a verb and a noun: it's the process we go through in the unseen world of human thought and emotion, and it is simultaneously the thing we want to give of ourselves to our patient. This precious thing, the thing that our patients come to us to receive from us—like satisfaction itself—exists in Einstein's quantum world. The process of delivering True Care happens in your heart and your mind, and it requires you to work with your own thoughts and emotions just like you work with your hands to start an IV or apply a bandage.

True Care, like all the best things in life, like the stuff that converts the physical building we call a house into the magical, warm, welcoming place we call a home, is the energy of love, connection, acceptance and belonging. All of this "stuff" is energy—packages or particles of quantum energy. These energies follow rules that are different from the rules that apply in Newton's world of dense matter, where we are used to living. Einstein's quantum world behaves very differently, and there are no absolutes; everything is relative. Here is a brief look at the difference between these two worlds, the world of matter and the world of energy.

Newton's Physical World	Einstein's Quantum World
Everything is linear	Everything is circular
Gravity and friction	Holographic universe / string theory
Time, space and motion	No time, space or motion (relative)
Physical five-sense reality	Multiple realities / parallel universes
Matter is the focus	Energy is the focus
Everything is dense / stagnant	Everything is fluid / dynamic

Tangible	Intangible
Seen	Unseen

"True Care" the noun, the thing we want to give to our patients, and "True Care" the verb, the active process we need to move through, both exist in this quantum world where we work with the intangible and unseen, where things are fluid and dynamic. Where everything is relative, there are no absolutes and two people in the same space can experience two different realities. Where everything is circular and energies travel through circuits, from one person to another and back again.

We are not dealing with the widgets of cure in the transaction of care. The transaction of care is a quantum transaction. It involves quantum commodities and deals with quantum energies, specifically energies of thought and emotion. So what is it that we are looking to exchange with our patient in the transaction of care? What are these unseen energies that we want to exchange?

In transactions in the physical world, it is very simple: you want x, you give money and they give you x. You want a car, you give the salesman your money and he gives you the car. You are the giver of money; he is the receiver of money. He is the giver of car and you are the receiver of car.

There is no money and there are no cars in the quantum world. In the quantum world, the transaction of care is the result of a simple perfect equation where the thing exchanged is a specific type of *energy*, in our case, True Care. There's a formula for this transaction that will always get you the good feeling you are looking for at work. This is the perfect equation you use to get what you want, always:

The **Perfect Equation**:

[We give **True Care**] + [Our patient receives **True Care**] = [**Quantum Satisfaction**]

This is the perfect energetic equation, our formula for success at work, the way we create job satisfaction, patient satisfaction and what I call the mutual satisfaction you generate for yourself and your patient in the quantum world of energy: Quantum Satisfaction, or satisfaction on both sides of the stethoscope.

When we give and our patient receives our True Care, the circuit of energy created effects a change in our patient and in us. Value is added to both parties, meaning and purpose are generated; both of our worlds are changed. This is the stuff you crave. This is your heart's desire as a hero of healthcare. This is your end game. This is what it is all about. This is what you were looking for when you came to this profession. This is the best part of your workday, and this is why you keep coming back for more. This is genuine, authentic and lasting Quantum Satisfaction.

No Strings Attached

If it is really this simple, why then is this not automatically happening already? What keeps the Perfect Equation from working? What I have learned is that our desire to care becomes corrupted over time. It gets deflected when we're told we have to keep our distance and rein in our compassion. And it begins to include other stuff, other demands and conditions attached to our desire to care.

Inside the energetic transaction of care, the giver and the receiver of care tend to want other things too, and they want exactly the same things or the exact opposites. While our wants may be the same or exactly opposite on either side of the stethoscope, our perception of our realities are vastly different as well.

The stuff patients want	The stuff we want
Respect	Respect
To have their symptoms relieved	To figure out their disease and diagnosis
To receive care (energy)	To provide them with a "cure" (a tangible thing)
To be cared for	To have patients care about their

	own health To decide who needs care To decide who deserves care To decide who is worthy of our care
Not to have to take responsibility for their situation or condition	Patients to take responsibility for their situation or condition
Things to happen in their time frame, on their schedule, at their convenience	Things to happen in our time frame; to decide who gets what and when
To blame the doctor or the hospital	To blame the patient
To be the customer who is always right	To be the authority who is always right
To feel that they are paying (or their insurance company is paying) for services, and thus demand that we care	To feel that we are doing them a favor, that our caring comes from the goodness of our hearts; we are here to deliver the "cure" and hand-holding is extra
To feel entitled, like they deserve	To feel entitled, like we deserve
The right to complain if they are not getting what they want	The right to complain if we are not getting what we want

By now, you should be able to see how we have become confused inside the transaction of care. We came here to care and make a difference, but we complain about lack of respect, appreciation, money and benefits. Our initial, simple, pure desire to care has become corrupted. We expect to give cure alone—a diagnosis, a minute of our time, a procedure, a drug, a test or an explanation—and we expect to get (or take) appreciation, respect, admiration or thanks. No wonder we don't feel good at work.

Because we are confused about the difference between care and cure, because we do not remember why we entered the transaction of care in the first place, there is clearly an imbalance between give and take in our current healthcare system. One of the problems is simple math. We expect to give one thing, say for example a diagnosis, and in exchange we would like to receive, or take, respect, appreciation, admiration and gratitude. We want to give one thing and get four things in exchange. What sense does that make? When you complete the transaction at the dealership, you give money and get a car. You don't give money and get a car, plus car insurance, plus free maintenance, plus a beautiful significant other to ride around in the front seat with you.

The real problem is one of currency. Do you notice that we want to give a thing (cure) and get an energy (appreciation) in return? It is sort of like going to the car dealer and expecting him to give you the car in exchange for your energy of loving everything about the car. We can't expect to trade physical things for energetic stuff. We all know money can't buy love. This is why we have to recalculate the transaction of care and formulate a new plan.

The biggest problem, though, has to do with the incongruence of our desires. You said you just want to give good healthcare, care that makes a difference for someone. In my research for this book, and in the previous chapters, it's been established that you chose this field because you want to care. **You said nothing about receiving anything in return**. Your simple desire to care has been corrupted. Now you have conditions that must be met before you can give care.

You will give care if and only if. You will give only if you get a thank you, respect or whatever it is that you have attached to your initial desire. By doing this, making this attachment, you have made your satisfaction dependent on another's behavior. How silly is that? We all know that we can't control the way others behave! In effect, you have given your power to create your own satisfaction away.

This sets you up to be a victim, a victim of another's incapacity for whatever reason to appreciate or thank you. Adam, the boy who taught us so much about satisfaction, did not thank the nurses at the pediatric hospital, he did not thank any of us, but we felt satisfaction simply because we helped him, we gave him another chance at life, we participated in a Lazarus case.

When you attach conditions to your care, or have expectations of others based on your giving care, your satisfaction is out of your own control. Why would anyone do this? The answer is simple. It is the easy way out. When you do this, you can blame your misery on everybody else. You no longer have to be responsible for your own satisfaction. You get to be a victim of everybody and everything. It seems really easy. But all you've really done is become the creator of your own dissatisfaction.

From this vantage point it is really simple to see why many of us are so miserable, why our current business-as-usual way of doing things just is not working. This is why so many of us are burned out, why so many of us are quitting, why so many of us feel resentment. This thinking that others should appreciate us, thank us, respect us—whatever the attachment we have in tow—is what corrupts our initial pure desire to care. This is what dooms us to failure.

When you enter the transaction of care with your attachments, you are really calculating, what's in it for me? With our attachments in tow, we have no concept of an even exchange. We have both unrealistic and scientifically impossible expectations. Why do you think so many people think that doctors and other people in healthcare are arrogant? Because we feel that once we give our cure, we should get the "thank you," the "oh, you are so great," the "wow, you saved my life." We also feel that we should get the raises, the perfect schedule and the flawless teamwork. We feel that we are entitled to so much for giving our cure.

We are doomed to a life of misery in healthcare if we do not all get this concept. If you give only so that you can get, you will never ever allow yourself to be the superhero you are destined to be. Think about what motivates a superhero: a new cape, front-page coverage in the *Daily Planet*, the bonus that pays for the exotic vacation, a raise so that they can afford the latest model of the Batmobile? None of these would matter to a superhero. The superhero knows that ultimate satisfaction lies in caring, making a difference, changing the world and saving the day.

This is the new formulation we have to come to. When we look for an energetic return for a physical action—when we expect satisfaction in exchange for delivering cure rather than care—we are disappointed. When it comes to energetic transactions, you can only exchange energy for energy. You cannot exchange physical goods or services for the energy of satisfaction. When we learn to give without expectation or attachments, without calculating what is in it for us, we will come to find that it is in the process of our giving that all of our needs and wants will be fulfilled.

Think about what happens when you give care, True Care, without calculating "what's in it for me?" When you give True Care and your patient feels your True Care, something happens for both of you, right then and there. Your patient feels better and you both finally exhale. Things seem to relax for a second or two. Then you can move on to delivering the technologies of cure in the most technically excellent way.

No matter what happens from this point forward for patients, they will always remember that moment they had with you, because of you. Whenever something like this happens, whenever we experience a special moment in time, we want to share the good news with everyone we know. That's why the patient will be quick to tell their family and loved ones about their good experience and you will be able to go home and say, *I had a great day at work.*

This moment you created is the place where Newton's laws of physical matter simply no longer apply. Newton's laws apply primarily to the cure. True Care exists in the quantum world where what you are feeling, what your patient is feeling, is what I call quantum satisfaction. Quantum laws apply to the energies you are both feeling, energies of thought and emotion. When your patient shares these energies with their family and their community, their family and their community will be feeling the same good feelings the patient felt as a result of you. They will spread the word about their good experience or the good experience of care their friend or their uncle had at your hospital.

You see, in the quantum world, things are not linear, and that feeling of satisfaction grows exponentially. If all these people who share in this feeling have a choice, they will pick your hospital as the one to come to when they need care in their search for a cure. As hospitals are surveying their patients about satisfaction with care, the "satisfaction scores" will improve. Your hospital will be rated higher and ultimately receive more compensation for the care delivered along with the cures. The hospital's bottom line will improve, the holes in the staffing schedule will improve, the equipment will be upgraded and you just might get a raise.

Now visits to your hospital for cures are up, simply because you are focused on and delivering True Care along with your cure. Your hospital administrator is happy, the board of directors and the hospitals investors are happy. The community begins to feel proud of your hospital. You begin to feel proud to work at your hospital. And people who have the same thoughts and feelings, the same consciousness around caring, that you do will be attracted to your facility because they will want to work alongside you, to be part of your team. They will want to be connected to your hospital that is clearly doing meaningful work, creating employee engagement, generating great outcomes and stellar measurable data and sending patient satisfaction scores through the roof. Your hospital will transform into a center of excellence that is focused on both care and cure.

To ignite this change, all we need to do as caregivers is to reconnect to our built-in desire to care, and to remember that we can create this quantum satisfaction if and only if we act from that pure and simple desire—if we stop confusing care with cure and execute the verb called True Care without any attachments. In order to generate quantum satisfaction, we have no choice but to care, for as we have already seen, we are hard-wired to care. Caring really does make us feel good.

Reversing Resentment

Did you hear that? If we want satisfaction, we have no choice but to care. We have to care. Nobody, and I mean nobody, likes *having* to do *anything*, especially when you don't feel good or you don't feel like it. We are already working so hard doing so many things, is it not obvious that we care? Doesn't everybody see our name badges and our uniforms?

It seems like we are practicing medicine in the Bermuda Triangle, where everything and anything mysteriously seems to go wrong, and everybody, and I do mean everybody, seems to be unhappy with what is going on. We feel we are doing everything we can to care about everyone and everything and, no matter how hard we work, "they" are telling us it's just not good enough. Then we take this personally and we hear society telling us that *we* are not good enough. As a result, we feel bad most of the time we are at work.

Many of us in this situation start to feel down and out. It is hard for us to see any value in what we do. All the paperwork and charting seems unnecessary for a trivial procedure. When it takes us more than twenty minutes to chart the encounter when someone comes in just to have their stitches removed, it feels like we are wasting our time. Even if we come to work with the best of intentions, in the best mood, we can lose it in a second in a drama with a patient or family member who acts out of frustration.

The crux of the problem, for those of us who have been working in healthcare for a while, as our own humanity is eroded over time by compassion fatigue and burnout, we naturally begin to resent the situation that we find ourselves in. You and I begin to resent the fact that our patients are not satisfied with our efforts, and this resentment separates us further from our original, simple, pure desire to care.

As caregivers, reconnecting to our original desire and taking action to fulfill that desire is what will bring us satisfaction. The big problem, however, is that in order to do this we will have to do the extremely hard work of rising above the resentment that we feel. How easy is it to move past or give up your resentment? This is never easy. And this is part of our recalculation process. I will teach you later how to effectively step over this hurdle. For now, just realize it is difficult to care when you don't feel like caring, and it is even more difficult to care when someone tells you that you have to care.

Patients come to us with a problem that they can't handle, and no matter how trivial it may seem to us, they are in a state of overwhelm and they want someone to care about them as well as cure them. They want someone to make it better for them. Through our work of remembering why we came here in the first place, connecting to our simple pure desire to care, and moving our resentment out of the way, we have shifted our position internally; when we act from this new place, we are able to move forward within the transaction of care so that both "needs"—our need to care and our patient's need to receive care—are fulfilled simultaneously.

It is quite simple, elegant and beautiful. But it is anything but easy. We think that our desire is enough. Our desire is not enough. Our delivery of a cure is not enough. We must establish the energetic circuitry that happens between the desire and its manifestation. Establishing this circuitry requires us to move through a process, to do work, to create or generate satisfaction. That's what the chapters ahead will help you do.

One realization that can make it easier for you in recalculating the transaction of care is to remember that you, the healthcare giver, are the one who consciously chose to be here. You are the willing participant. The patient did not make a conscious choice to be sick or need your help. The patient is only there, right in front of you, to give you the opportunity to fulfill your original desire. The patient was not born to be sick. You were born to care. Remembering this will make it easier for you to recalculate things so that you no longer *have to* care, but *want to* care.

This is a perfect setup for the Perfect Equation. We can now begin to recalculate our position so that we can see the patient not as an obstacle, but as a gift. If you did not have this angry, disgruntled, entitled patient in front of you, you would not be in a position to "get" satisfaction.

Society has raised the bar for us: not only do we have to put our own personal needs, wants and desires aside in order to execute the delivery of True Care, but now we have to do the additional, extremely difficult work of moving past our resentment, and looking past our patient's bad behavior, to see the hurting human who is suffering right in front of us, in order to get to the place where we actually want to give care to him. While resentment may seem like a strong word, remember the effects of compassion fatigue and burnout are even more strongly felt here, when it is oh so difficult to be caring.

As a result of our personal and collective secondary PTSD, we as care givers are working with both physical and emotional exhaustion. Our ability to feel empathy for our patients and our co-workers has been greatly diminished over time. We have become irritable and quick to anger. We have become cynical, especially at work. We have over time lost our concern or respect for other people and our perceptions of people have become dehumanized. We label people or groups of people in a derogatory manner and we dread working with certain types of patients or certain patients in particular.

That is a whole lot of stuff to move out of the way or rise above in order to generate and deliver True Care for another. The big bonus for us is that when we do all of this hard work, when we turn the situation around, when we are the cause in this new scenario, when we make things better for our patient, we not only get to feel good—we get to feel incredibly good, beyond-our-wildest-expectations good. Generating compassion for our more difficult patients erases years of the effects of burnout in our own emotional systems and neurologic anatomy.

We forget we came here because we wanted to care, and we confuse the delivery of cure, physical goods and services, with the energetic action of giving care. Our resentment comes from the facts that we forgot we came to care, we have confused cure and care, and now we know that for all those years we believed that connecting was bad for us and our patients, True Care actually requires us to get close and connect to our patients. Reconnecting to our original desire to care changes that feeling of resentment, and this changes everything, because now we "**get to**" rather than "have to" care. When you feel like you have to, you feel like a slave. Naturally you're resentful! When you get to, you are free and you are in control. You actually want to find creative ways to care. You are the cause. You are the creator of your own fulfillment.

The work you have to do is not really the caring. It is always easy to care, once you can get past the distractions and the resentments and remember that's why you're here. For the most part, the caring is fairly straightforward. The work you have to do is removing the roadblocks and barriers that are in the way of your caring. The work you have to do is to get yourself clear enough to care. You have to become **clear to care**.

Reclaiming Your Power

By now we should all have come to the understanding that what we really want is to derive our own personal satisfaction from caring. If you do not see this by now, you might as well stop reading; there will be no solution for you. If you want to argue with me that what you really need to feel satisfaction is a new job or a different patient, that you really do have an awful boss, that you need someone to fix the medical system, that you need a better economy, that you need to live in a better society, that you are a victim of your circumstances, well, then set the book down and go back to your misery.

You are not wrong. You are right. The system *is* broken, the economy and society *are* a mess. You are often being mistreated by the very people that you are trying to help. Your feelings are valid. **The circumstances we operate in today are totally messed up—but what you have to understand is that you, and only you, are responsible for your own happiness, regardless of your circumstances**.

In order to feel happy, you have to let go of the idea that you are a victim. If you are going to be a modern hero of healthcare, if you are going to change the world and save the day, you can never lay blame for your unhappiness, your ineffectiveness or your inability to create satisfaction for yourself on anyone or anything outside yourself. Victims are powerless to feel good. That is why they complain, because they want others to feel sorry for them. We must all let go of our victim mentality. We must reclaim our power.

Our power is the power to feel good, to be the cause of a new and better reality, not only for ourselves but for our patients, their families, the hospital, our co-workers, our community and our society. We have the power to make things better, to ease the pain, to mitigate the suffering, to help and to heal. The reason we have this power is because we were born with a built-in, altruistic, pure and simple desire to care.

When we all come to consensus and understand that no one will solve our problems for us, that we must be the change we want to see in this world, we will finally understand just how powerful each and every one of us is. We are intelligent, probably hyper-intelligent; we are resilient and we are energetic. We feel we were born to or called to do this work. We already have everything we need to be successful. We have only one problem: all the chaos we swim in has left us confused about what is really going on.

We have thought and believed that we will have satisfaction if and only if the rest of the world changes. Now we embrace the knowledge that when we face a challenge, when we find it difficult to care, the only way we can get the satisfaction we seek is to change ourselves. This change we must undergo is internal—it involves our thoughts and our feelings—and to change internally is to transform in the quantum world. **Once we have transformed ourselves, we can transcend our previous limits, and we most definitely have the power to be truly effective givers of care, and that changes everything**.

Think of it like the process Superman used. Whenever he heard the call to action, he had to stop and drop everything he was doing and run into a phone booth to change. When we hear the call to action, when we feel ourselves getting angry or we begin to feel resentful and we actually don't want to care, when we would rather act out in a negative way, we must stop and drop everything we are doing and run inside our heads, run inside our hearts, and change internally, inside the quantum reality. Unlike Superman, our appearance won't change, but changing our thoughts and feelings will allow us to see past all the distractions, all the chaos, and see that the one in front of us needs our care.

From this new place within, we will be able to use our quantum powers of thought and emotion to find the way to care, regardless of the situation or circumstance, and this is our quantum power to be the cause of change in this world. Our work is to use our quantum thoughts and emotions, our knowledge, our wisdom and our perspective, to transform ourselves into the healers we were born to be and become the heroes of modern healthcare we are destined to become.

If you get this, then I can't wait to move on, because this is the most difficult part of our transformation from zeros to heroes. The rest is simple, and I am about to give you your silver bullet, the bullet that will slay any dragon that stands between you and your desire to care.

Chapter 6

The TIME OUT Tool

We have covered quite a lot of ground so far. At the risk of being redundant, I need to make certain that you are with me. We are traveling on a journey, the healthcare hero's journey to the land of quantum satisfaction, and by this point you should be seeing your world and your place in it very differently. You should be starting to realize that there most definitely is a way that we can feel better at work and, more importantly, we hold the key to making it happen.

How did we get here? Let's review. We came to healthcare because we had a pure and simple desire to care—to help people feel better. It took years of training for us to finally get to their bedsides, and in that time we began, quite naturally, to mistake *cure* for *care*. Because we focused all our attention on cure, we got really good at it, yet our patients weren't happy—they saw us as arrogant and uncaring. Because we were working so hard to deliver their cures, this really hurt! Now, no matter how hard we try, we can't seem to satisfy our patients, so we grow weary and resentful and we start to burn out, which just makes it that much harder to care. As a result, nobody's desires are being fulfilled on either side of the stethoscope.

But there is hope, and we've already taken several steps in the direction of renewed satisfaction, fulfillment and joy in our work. Let's look again at the steps so far:

1. Now you **REMEMBER** what you came here for in the first place, and you've reconnected to your desire to care, to make a difference, to make patients feel better *because* you care.

2. You know that no one can give satisfaction to you. You know that only you can **EARN** your satisfaction for yourself. You've realized that you are responsible for creating your own satisfaction, and if you are going to feel good, you have to shift your focus from the physical components of cure to the intangible energies of care.

3. You have learned to **FORMULATE** your plan for getting the satisfaction you crave that comes from caring. You have recalculated the transaction of care according to the Perfect Equation, by which your giving True Care and your patient's receiving your True Care add up to the energy of satisfaction in the quantum world of thought and emotion. You have learned to free yourself from your (hidden) attachments or agenda.

4. Now it's time to reframe your role in the patient encounter and your position in regards to your goal: to understand that the obstacles to your satisfaction aren't outside you, but within you. Here you will **LOOK** at your position within the transaction of care and ask yourself if you are the *cause* of something better or the *effect* of another's situation. You will learn to ask yourself, am I reacting or am I responding?

Physics and the Patient Encounter

We can all feel good and make our patients feel better while delivering all the marvelous and miraculous technological goods and services we already have to offer. The question that remains is how. The answer lies in knowing that in order to feel good about the cure we are delivering, we also have to be the cause of our patient's feeling better, always, no exceptions. We can never be the effect of our situation, our broken system, our past failures, our own burnout, or our patient's anger.

Normally, when people interact, the person who speaks first is the cause and the one who reacts is the effect. The key to understanding how we can become the cause lies inside the interpersonal encounter, or what we call the patient encounter at work. The key to understanding *this*, in turn, lies in the rules that govern energy exchange between two humans. There are dynamics in action, when the energies of thought and emotion interact, that we must understand if we are going to use our thoughts and emotions to create change in our patients in ways that will cause them to feel better. For a long time we have been ill equipped to discuss the way our thoughts and emotions can interact with another's in any encounter, let alone the patient encounter. Thanks to Einstein's insight into the quantum world, we can now develop a model for understanding this dynamic, a vocabulary for talking about it and, most importantly, a tool kit for repairing it.

So what am I really talking about? For an answer, we need to explore a little more the difference between Newtonian physics and quantum mechanics.

Sir Isaac Newton wrote three laws that describe the motion of objects in our physical world. These three laws make up the bulk of what we know about classical mechanics, which explain and predict the motion of dense matter or physical objects. These laws have guided scientists for the past three centuries. Here is my best attempt to summarize them.

The first law is responsible for the popular expression "Bodies at rest tend to stay at rest and bodies in motion tend to stay in motion." This law states that every physical body remains in a state of rest or uniform motion with constant velocity, unless it is acted upon by an external force that creates an imbalance. This means that in the absence of such a force, a body's center of mass either remains at rest or moves at a constant speed in a straight line.

His second law is expressed $F = ma$. This law states that a body of mass (m) subject to a force (F) undergoes an acceleration (a) that has the same direction as the force and a magnitude that is directly proportional to the force and inversely proportional to the mass. You could say the concept of entropy is born here, where decay in these systems is inevitable. Left unattended, these systems disorganize into chaos.

His third law is the most important to those of us who want to be healthcare heroes. It states that the mutual forces of action and reaction between two bodies of mass are equal, opposite and co-linear. Get this loud and clear, please: this means that, whenever a first body of mass exerts a force (F) on a second body of mass, the second body must exert a force (-F) that is equal and in opposition. This law is sometimes stated this way: "For every action, there is an equal and opposite reaction."

This third law of Isaac Newton's is what allowed NASA to put a man on the moon. This law is very important to space travel—and just as important to our journey toward satisfaction. We really need to understand this law if we want to become successful at caring for others, if we want to become heroes to our patients, if we want our patients and ourselves to feel good again.

If you push on something, it pushes back on you. That is why, if you lean on a wall, you don't just fall through it. The wall pushes back on you. The harder you push on the wall, the harder it pushes back on you, and this is why neither of you moves. You both stay in place.

If you throw an object, the harder you throw it, the harder it will push back on you. In theory, you should both be moving away from each other, but this is hard to see most of the time, because the friction between you and the ground keeps you in place while the thing you threw travels away from you. But if you were to put on a pair of roller skates and then throw something, you and the thing you threw would both move away from each other (in opposite directions). The bigger the push, the bigger the push back—this is why cannons and guns recoil.

You should be starting to realize that this law applies to human interaction as well. To prove it to yourself, stop reading and go find a person to help you. Don't tell them what you want to do, just ask them to face you. You place your right palm against their left palm and just stand there for a second or two. Then gently start to push against their hand. Then push a little harder . . . see what happens. When you push, they push back. When you push harder, they push back harder. The bigger the push, the bigger the push back.

But when we are inside the patient encounter, executing the transaction of care according to the perfect equation, we're working with our thoughts and emotions, which are not dense physical matter. So what laws apply here? We now have to look to Albert Einstein for help.

Einstein's Theory of Relativity is used to derive the rules that apply to stuff in the unseen, intangible world, the quantum world, where satisfaction exists. Einstein's theory modifies Newtonian mechanics so that we get a new set of rules or laws, called quantum mechanics. Quantum mechanics describes the behavior of those things that we do not have the ability or the sensory apparatus to perceive.

The game-changing insight Einstein brought to the table is encapsulated in the famous formula $E = mc^2$ (where E is energy, m is mass, and c is the speed of light in a vacuum). Energy and matter cannot be created or destroyed, only changed from one form to the other (and back again), and they exist not as separate entities, but on a continuum.

Matter can affect energy, as is proved by Einstein's work with the speed of light. He discovered that this speed is constant, whether it comes from a moving source such as a speeding car's headlights or a stationary source like a ceiling light—but only in a vacuum, a place where there is no physical matter. The vast emptiness of space is such a place, and the speed of light is constant there. Here on earth, where we practice medicine, light can be slowed, reflected or refracted by physical matter: matter affecting energy. And energy can affect matter: heat makes water boil and turn into steam; microwaves cook food.

Clinically, it should be obvious that energy can affect matter. Do we not use electricity to jump-start the heart, and does not that electricity, if not properly grounded, sometimes char the tissues? Our thoughts and our emotions are energies, so they too can affect physical matter, and this is reflected in our patients when their faces relax, their blood pressure falls, their pulses slow and they finally exhale that deep breath of satisfaction.

Reaction and Response

We can learn quite a bit about our situation at the bedside in healthcare today by observing a simple toy that illustrates how perpetual motion machines work. You know what I am talking about—those metal balls suspended on V-shaped wires hanging from a frame. When you lift a ball at one end and release it, it strikes the next ball, and one ball at the other end flies up to the same height. If you lift two balls, two balls at the other end fly up: an equal and opposite reaction. Yet these desktop toys, like all perpetual-motion machines, because of Newton's laws of thermodynamics and Einstein's laws of quantum physics, always come to a standstill. Without some energy being added to the system, friction will cause it to lose energy and its movement to decay.

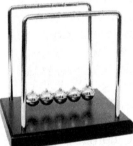

If these steel balls could make the choice to inject more energy, this machine could run forever, not lose energy over time, not decay and ultimately stop. However, these little steel balls don't have the free will to do that. These little steel balls of dense physical matter can only react.

Inside the human encounter, the patient encounter, there are two dense physical bodies, but the situation is more complex: these two bodies, you and your patient, also contain and transmit all sorts of energies, and these have the power to influence each other. These energies are thoughts mingled with emotion. They are the energies of satisfaction, fear, compassion, anger, denial, tolerance, empathy and such. If we as healthcare providers are going to give True Care, a specific blend of energies, we must be able to stop or interrupt the action-reaction cycle and inject these energies into the system.

Please pay attention here: this next concept is of paramount importance to your transformation from feeling bad, to feeling good at work. The little steel balls in our perpetual-motion machine have no choice but to react. Humans do have the option to respond rather than react!

A hungry cat, when confronted with a mouse, has no choice but to pounce. The cat automatically reacts. There is no conscious thought that goes into the cat's reaction. We as humans have free will. When we automatically react to another human's bad behavior, or even their good behavior, we are functioning on the level of our own personal animal within.

If we want to be the cause instead of the effect, it is necessary that we not behave like animals and automatically react. We must subdue our personal beast within, our automatic physiologic reaction, and take the option to respond instead. The reality is that, whether or not we have been aware of it, by not making a conscious choice in any situation we are always reacting, and therefore we are always the effect rather than the cause. When we choose, we become proactive rather than reactive, this choice to respond gives us the opportunity to be the cause of something different.

Response is very different from reaction. Response requires us to exercise our free will. Response requires us to interrupt the action-reaction cycle, just for a second, and inject the energies of thought and emotion into the human-human interaction. A reaction is automatic and animal-like. A response is well thought out and full of the positive energies contained within our concept of True Care. We add our benevolent energies of kindness, tolerance, understanding, empathy and compassion to the system of human interpersonal interaction, and this allows us to impart the energies of positive thoughts and emotions to the other, to be the cause of a change for the other, to make things better for one another.

This is how we will look at our position inside the transaction of care: we use this information to understand that along with being a giver of care comes the need to be the cause of something better. Activating our free will is what will allow us to take our control back in any situation. Activating our free will, by absolutely refusing to react, is what interrupts that action-reaction cycle. Once this cycle is interrupted, we use our free will to inject positive benevolent energies, and now we become the cause. Taking the option to respond is what allows us to be the cause within any interpersonal exchange or encounter.

By stopping the action-reaction cycle even just for a split second, we create the space to inject our wisdom, knowledge and understanding coupled with the positive emotions of tolerance, kindness, compassion, empathy and concern. Once we have injected these good quantum energies into the system, we can respond. With this quantum energy added to the delivery of our cure, we will change the dynamics in the system, change what the patient is feeling and change the way his body is functioning, and he will feel both emotionally and physically better. Think of it like a shot of medicine. You inject the pain medicine into a patient's system, it causes a change in the way his body is functioning and the pain is eased. Here, however we are injecting positive thought and emotional energy (the energetic substance of True Care, the noun) into our energetic interaction (the energetic process of True Care, the verb) with our patient; this changes the way their thoughts and emotions are functioning, and their emotional pain is eased, and we earn our own satisfaction and feel good.

Slaying the Dragons

Now, there is one more giant piece of the puzzle you have to understand. In Newton's world, the world of *cure*, the problem is usually obvious and so is the solution. If the patient has no heartbeat, you must start CPR. If the patient is bleeding, you must stop the bleeding. If there is a splinter in her foot, you must remove the splinter. Easy.

In Einstein's world, the world of *care*, the problem is never the problem, especially as it relates to action-reaction, the cause and the effect, in the uniquely human interaction. Humans are not inanimate, unthinking little balls just bouncing off one another, although we behave as such when we automatically react rather than stopping to engage a thinking, feeling response. Humans are a complex blend of the physical (biological matter, chemical equations and electrical processes), the emotional (feelings) and the mental (thoughts), all blending together to determine the state of the organism. It is important to understand that each of these elements is of a higher order than the next: the emotional is of a higher order than the physical, and the mental is of a higher order than the emotional.

When we automatically react, we reverse the order and let our emotions generate our thoughts, which in turn generate our words and actions. This is how the cat catches the mouse. Thoughts, however, being of a higher order than emotions, can control emotions, generate different emotions. When we respond, we must use a *thought* to generate the *emotions* we will add to the thought to generate the quantum substance we now know as True Care. This is the quantum stuff that we will inject into our encounter with our patient. Taking the time to stop, think and inject into the patient encounter a different positive thought to generate positive emotions within us—this gives us the power we need to always be the cause of something better, something better than what was or what is. During our interactions with patients and each other, we can always look at our position and ask, am I the cause or am I the effect? This will help us to know if we are reacting or responding. The goal is to always take the option to respond.

It is really that simple, but, as usual, it is not that easy to identify the obstacles, those thoughts that get in the way of us exercising our free will to achieve our ultimate desire of care. Earlier we talked about feeling resentful. Why would anyone feel resentment in the first place? It is because all humans live with something called memory. We remember, consciously or unconsciously, every time we have been hurt, felt embarrassed, or failed. We have all sorts of worries and fears that we carry around with us like baggage. All humans do this, caregivers and patients alike. Most of the time we are not even aware of what the specific negativity is that we are carrying around with us.

It is this baggage we carry that causes us to unconsciously react rather than take the option to respond. We see situations through our own particular lens, which is not clear, but clouded with our fears, wounds and failures. Because of this, we are like an animal being threatened, and our emotions, our amygdala and our limbic system in the lower regions of our brain take control away from our higher cortex. When we react, we are just the effect of our environment, our situation, our patient or their family member—and totally ineffective as caregivers. We cannot be the cause of something better when we react.

This is why, in the quantum world, when it comes to the patient interaction, the problem is never the problem. The problem is our automatic reaction. Our automatic reaction, shaped by our past, is the one thing that keeps us separated from our desire to care and make a difference for another. We will speak volumes about this in the next chapters of the book, but for right now, we need a tool—something we can use to stop our automatic reaction. Something that will allow us to use our free will to inject a thought or emotion, which will allow us to inject the quantum energies of True Care, which will allow us to change things for our patient so that we can both feel better.

Shutting Down Our Automatic Reaction

The tool you want to reach for in any difficult situation is the **TIME OUT** tool. This tool, when you use it, will always allow you to generate a thinking, feeling, compassionate, and empathetic response that will effectively generate the True Care that changes everything. When you look at your position inside the patient encounter and the transaction of care, and you realize that you are the effect and not the cause, this silver bullet will take down every dragon in your path—every obstacle of resentment, anger or fear—and let you transform yourself to become someone's healthcare hero. Here is how the **TIME OUT** tool works.

1. A situation occurs. As you're reacting to it, **<u>STOP</u>**, recognize your automatic reaction and stop yourself.

2. **REALIZE** that the situation is not the obstacle; the obstacle is your reaction to the situation, your reactive thoughts and emotions that are getting in the way of your giving True Care.

3. **IDENTIFY** the reactive thoughts and emotions inside you and choose to inject new thoughts and emotions that match your desire to give True Care.

4. Now **SPEAK** or **ACT** from this new internal quantum reality and effectively give your True Care.

Understanding the TIME OUT Tool

The Perfect Equation is simple, but it is not easy. That's why we need the **TIME OUT** tool. We now are clear that we cannot have any personal (hidden) attachments to our giving care, no unspoken demand for appreciation, respect or a thank you. Ours can be a thankless job, and that's okay, because the thank you pales in comparison to the inner feeling that swells up within us when we act compassionately and heroically—there truly is nothing better for us. But as heroes we are still human.

We have human feelings too, but our feelings, when they are part of an automatic reaction, get in our way. This is why we need the **TIME OUT** tool. The **TIME OUT** tool allows us to use the power of our mind to cut out or remove the thoughts and emotions that arise from our automatic biologic physical reaction and inject new thoughts from our mind that change the neurochemistry in our prefrontal cortex that then allows us to effectively become the cause inside the transaction of care. When we are effective at injecting new thoughts that will allow us to create the satisfaction we crave, we know beyond a shadow of a doubt that it is because of us, because of what we are thinking, feeling, saying and doing, that our patient experiences something better, that we ourselves experience something better, that we ourselves get better and recover from compassion fatigue and burnout.

There is only one thing that stands between us and giving care. That thing is inside us. That thing is a piece of our mammalian physiology and our emotions, contained within our amygdala and limbic system, including our past experiences and memories stored there. If we are already emotionally wounded by the secondary PTSD of compassion fatigue and burnout, those negative emotions and thoughts can be very loud and difficult to overcome. When we are challenged to give care, when we are thinking and feeling that we don't want to for whatever reason, we have to dump our negative thoughts and feelings and mindfully inject new, positive thoughts and feelings that put us in a different internal quantum space, that change the neurochemistry in our brains and bodies. In order to give care, we have to identify our negative thoughts and feelings and move them out of our own way. To do this, we reach for our one and only surefire tool, the **TIME OUT** tool.

This tool is what will allow us to create the inner transformation we need to become the cause, rather than the effect, in our encounters. It will allow us to put our own baggage down long enough to clear our mind and reconnect to our heart's original desire to care. From this place where we are clear about what we really want, we can inject new thoughts and emotions into the encounter so that we become the cause of our patient's feeling better.

When we have gone through our personal inner transformation (the significant change in our internal, neurochemical, biological state) by injecting new consciousness, we go from having almost no ability to care, to being ready, willing and able to care. **It is always easy to care when you are clear to care.** We can then see the hurting human in front of us and share our own new, more powerful thoughts and emotions with him or her. These will be thoughts and feelings that our patient has the capacity to receive, and these will change their world and save our day.

We, the givers of care, are the ones who actually benefit the most from taking the TIME OUT. We will never be effective when we leave the autopilot on—when we automatically react, rather than stopping the automatic reaction with the **TIME OUT** tool. Only when we take the option to take the **TIME OUT**, in order to create a thinking and feeling response, will we be able to inject the energies of True Care into our interaction with another and be the cause of our own satisfaction when our prefrontal cortex lights up in the altruistic state of compassion. This feeling good is actually the result of the neurochemistry we create in our own brains.

As I was about to write this chapter for you, I found myself in just such a situation—not with a patient, but with a colleague. You see, there was this doctor whom I found to be extremely challenging. My last contact with him had been a couple of weeks earlier when he was relieving me at 7 a.m. after a very demanding ten-hour night shift. He was about twenty-five minutes late and he had not bothered to call and let us know. When he finally did show up, he offered no excuse and extended no apology.

Test results came back on one of the patients I had planned to turn over to him in the time we were waiting for him to arrive, and he had the gall to ask me to stay over even longer to make disposition and close the encounter with this patient. I said nothing to him, but I was seething inside. I saw him as arrogant, lazy and uncaring. I felt taken advantage of, I felt disrespected, I was angry. I already knew that he was not my problem. My problem was my reactive anger and feelings of being disrespected. In spite of the fact that I knew that MY anger was MY problem, I just could not find a way out of that negativity. I carried this anger with me until I saw him at work again

This time I was working alongside him. During our shift, he never had more than two or three patients on the board at any one time, and it was busy. I felt like I was carrying the whole department. Near the end of his shift, he held on to two patients and did not see anyone else for two hours—until three minutes after his shift was over, when he picked up a new patient with a complicated problem. He then milked the clock for another forty-five minutes and turned that patient over to me so he could leave. My distain for him grew to horrible proportions of resentment. Again, I felt disrespected, taken advantage of and angry.

Feeling these emotions and having these thoughts was especially a problem for me because I was working clinically. When we are preoccupied with these sorts of negative thoughts and emotions, it is extremely difficult to move into the internal quantum space where it is possible to really care for others. The problem was that I was working, caring for patients, looking for satisfaction inside each and every patient encounter, and my resentment was making it even more challenging.

I did not directly confront him and ask him to pull his fair share of the load, first and foremost because I had done this many other times with many other doctors and it never turned out well. Second, because I was angry and it is never good to confront another when you are angry—it's best to wait a few days and let the emotional charge dissipate. Third, I realize that everyone in this profession is suffering from some degree of burnout, and asking someone who suffers from the effects of PTSD to be reasonable is not really a sound idea. If they could do better, they would already be doing better. So I kept my thoughts and feelings to myself.

I resisted the urge to lash out at the other doctor, the urge to trash talk about him to the staff, the urge to chastise him, shame and humiliate him publicly. But my resentment of the situation was clearly standing in between me and another amazing, fulfilling day at work. Worse yet, I knew that. Knowledge is power, but it did not give me the power I needed at that moment to step around or rise above the resentment and anger I was feeling. Even worse, I was writing a book to help you feel better and I found myself feeling just as bad as I had seven or eight years ago, when I was so bitter that I had to quit my job.

As I left work that morning, I was full of venom, poison and righteous indignation. However, I knew beyond a shadow of a doubt that "that doctor" was not the problem. Remember, in the quantum world of thoughts and emotions, in the quantum world of satisfaction, the problem is never the problem. The problem was me, or rather, my reaction to that particular doctor. What was I holding on to? What was it that I refused to let go of? What was it inside me that prevented me from lifting myself out of my reactive thoughts and emotions?

I thought about how I should be grateful that I could care for so many patients simultaneously. I thought about how I should feel thankful and blessed that I had the capacity to do so. But no matter how hard I tried, I could not let go. I could not rise above my garbage thoughts about this doctor and all the negative emotions these powerful thoughts were causing me to feel. I actually started to feel like this whole book was a waste of time. I had to, just had to, resolve this—not only for me, but for you.

I've told you that the **TIME OUT** tool always works, never fails, that it is your silver bullet, that it will slay any dragon that stands between you and your personal satisfaction, at work or in life. Here I was, having successfully applied step one and step two: I had stopped myself, and I had realized that it was my own automatic thoughts and feelings that were standing in my way.

I was even able to complete the first part of step three: I had successfully identified the negative thoughts and feelings; I had named them, explored them and understood them. But I was not yet able to replace them with new thoughts that would generate the words and behaviors that would allow me to feel my own satisfaction. I was stuck. Yet I knew this formula always worked. It had to work for me now, or I had to scrap the entire book.

What was my righteous indignation all about? Well, I was clearly standing in judgment of this doctor. He was an ass. He was arrogant. He was lazy. He was uncaring. He took advantage of people, me included. He would throw his own mother under the bus if it made his life just a little easier. He was pathetic and disgusting. Worse yet, when I asked others at work, "What do you think about him?" they said the same things. So I was right, damn it!

But I want to be happy—who cares if I am right? What good is being right if I am miserable? So, looking for the way out of my negative quantum space, I dug deeper. Follow me here. I've already realized that I am standing in judgment of that doctor. The only reason I should stand in judgment of another is what? It is extremely difficult to admit, but the truth is that if I judge him as bad, I can see myself as good.

There are two obvious problems with this thought process. First, when I make him the bad guy, I become a victim of his behavior, the effect. He is the cause. If I am going to be happy at work and in life, I always have to be the cause of my own satisfaction and happiness. Second, when I stand in judgment of another, making him wrong, I am projecting my thoughts, my essence and my opinions on him, even though I know nothing about him, what his understanding of life is, what baggage he carries with him. I know that judging him so that I can feel better about myself never works. I know that my judging him only dooms me to a dark reality that it is almost impossible to escape.

It was from this perspective that I was able to ask myself, *Who is the worse doctor of the two, him or me?* I knew the answer: me. I knew better, I had tools, I had perspective, I already had the map to nirvana, but I was stubbornly refusing to use them. Why? Because I am stubborn, that's why. We are all stubborn in this respect. This is just a stupid game that our beast within plays with us, keeping us stuck in the mud of resentment, hatred and smoldering anger.

I thought to myself, *I am sick of being the bigger man, the one who does the right thing, the one who takes the high road, the nice guy who finishes last. Why doesn't that doctor just do the right thing?* But then I also thought, *I am so sick of this. I am so tired of hurting myself, blocking my own joy with these stupid attachments and baggage. I am so sick and tired of being the effect, I so desperately want to be the cause, and as long as I play this game, I am doomed to be stuck in the mud—I will never soar like an eagle.*

That was all it took: I decided to step out of the game. No more. No more waiting for that doctor to change in order for me to feel good. He is doing what he does and I need to do what I do. There is nothing wrong with him and nothing right with me. There is nothing to change externally. The only thing I have to do is change internally.

Remember that our beast within is actually our limbic system and amygdala; it is our built-in automatic physiology and neurochemistry. It is based on thousands of years of evolution and contains within it the memory of every time we were ever hurt, embarrassed or otherwise harmed by another in our whole life. In medicine and nursing, our amygdala and limbic system contain all the negative memories of each time we were hurt by one of our colleagues, our patients or a family member—this memory is part and parcel of our emotional wounding, the PTSD of compassion fatigue and burnout. These automatic physiologic mechanisms are designed to keep us safe, but not necessarily happy or satisfied. It will require heroic, mindful effort to rise above this powerful machinery of ours, which is designed to alert us to situations that can hurt us again.

The only way to rise above our automatic physiology is to become conscious of what is really happening and then use the thoughts in our mind to change the chemistry in our brain. I had come to the place where I realized that allowing this automatic loop to run unconsciously was really hurting me and limiting me. It was my desire to let it go that allowed me to come to the realization that I have no choice but to do more, because I have the capacity to do more, and the more I do, the harder I work, the more satisfaction, joy, happiness and peace of mind I can create for myself and share with others.

Earlier, I showed you that we have no choice but to care, because caring is built right into our DNA as caregivers. Caregiving is what turns us on, excites us and ignites our passion. Caregiving is what makes us fully alive. This hard-won lesson will set you free as it did me. Seeing this clearly allowed me to see that my judgment of others really only hurts me, blocks me, stifles me and diminishes me. My judgment of others, even if I am right, only limits me. My judgment of others only makes me less than them, lower than them, worse than them, unhappier, more frustrated and less satisfied than them, even if I am right. When I focus on judging others, I cut myself off from life itself, all the goodness, all the sweetness; all the best life has to offer. I am no masochist. I am not going to play that game.

Armed with these new quantum thoughts and emotions, I prepared myself to go back to work, with the same doctor, in the same circumstances. I had finally completed step three of the **TIME OUT** tool. I had put myself in a new quantum space. I had successfully changed my own neurochemistry with my own thoughts.

I walked into the department with these new realizations, ready to execute step four of the **TIME OUT** tool, to reframe my position as the cause rather than the effect, to speak and act from my own new positive personal quantum reality and give True Care from there. The minute I walked through the ambulance bay into the department, I saw to my surprise that that doctor, the bad guy, the one I stood in judgment of, well, he was not there. There was a man who looked just like him, who was wearing his lab coat and name badge, but it seemed to me as if he was totally transformed. He was seeing lots of patients now, he was reaching out to me, it was clear that he was trying to befriend me.

This shift was even busier than the last two, but things just seemed to flow, the rest of the staff seemed more energetic, we experienced flawless teamwork. The charge nurse who likes to blame my ADD for the fact that there are so many patients in the department—she was actually working hard, expediting things, supporting her nurses and techs in a way I did not even know she was capable of. The staff seemed genuinely happy to be working and, better yet, to be working with each other.

I was wondering, *Am I dreaming? Have I died and gone to heaven? How could this be, that the change in me changed my world, and the world of everyone that I work with, and the patients we care for, and the hospital?* This is our power, our superhuman healthcare hero power, to change the world and save the day. I knew for certain that this was no dream when that doctor, that awful doctor, asked me if there was anything he could do to help me before he left at the end of his shift. He left by shaking my hand and saying good night, and he had a smile on his face instead of a scowl.

I realize now, more than ever before, that this book, my gift to all of you, is not something that I want to do, this is something I *have* to do, for the only way I can get more satisfaction is to do more, to be more, to be the one who cares to change the world and show you how to do the same. I have to take responsibility, as we all do, for lifting those we work with, live with and struggle with to higher ground, to a new reality where we can all get clear enough to care. Not because it is the right thing to do, but because this is the only way we can all be good, do good and feel good every day of our working lives.

The Good, the Bad, and the Entitled

My problem with that doctor made it hard for me to give care to any of my patients until I used the **TIME OUT** tool to shift into a new quantum space. Let's look at what happens when you're face to face with *one* difficult patient. You may think the patient is rude, arrogant, not sick enough to need you, and carrying around a huge chip on his or her shoulder. And you may be right in your assessment. But holding on to being right is the very thing that you are going to have to move out of the way if you want to be satisfied.

So what if your patient is a jerk? Does that mean that you suddenly can't care for him? Think about it, jerks cut you off in traffic and give you the finger on your way to work. These same jerks are in car accidents, they have heart attacks, and they have strokes every day. When these jerks come into the Emergency Department, they need your care. They certainly were not born with a desire to be your patient, but you were born with a desire to care. You *chose* to be the one who cares.

When these jerks are in a serious car accident, when it is life or death, when every second counts, suddenly neither you nor I think about whether or not our patient is a jerk. It's clear that they need our care, jerk or saint; there is a really hurting human in front of us, and what we do right now matters! That is what is so great about stepping inside the emergency. When we are inside the emergency, as with Adam, all of our distractions, our opinions, our feelings about them fall away. Our primary, uncorrupted desire to care takes over and we are moved into our heroic selves automatically. In these extreme situations, we need none of the wisdom, perspective, tools or framework I have included in this book. All of it happens automatically because our desire to care, our desire to be the one who makes a difference, is so intense and all-consuming. When we step inside the emergency it is so simple to care. But what happens when there is no emergency to step inside, and there is that jerk in front of us, demanding our care? What happens then?

When the jerk is brought in by EMS in cardiac arrest, the fact that he's a jerk is not a problem. When the same jerk shows up at 3 a.m. with a cough but no fever, or a discharge from his penis, suddenly it *is* a problem. Everything that bothers you, challenges you, irritates or otherwise disturbs you in your environment triggers something inside you, and that something inside you is the real obstacle to your satisfaction. That something inside you is your automatic physiologic reaction. Yes, you may be right that the patient is rude; you may have the right to be irritated and annoyed. But being right in this situation doesn't work if you are going to successfully give care, to feel empathy, to turn on your own compassion, to be the cause of the patient feeling better. Holding on to being right will only leave you feeling trapped, frustrated, drained and exhausted. By choosing to be right instead of choosing to inject True Care, you are choosing your unsatisfied reality.

There is one particular situation we encounter with patients several times a day, each and every day. *Entitlement* makes it exceptionally difficult for us to move our negative thoughts and feelings out of the way of our caring. In today's society, we all feel entitled to something. Almost all of us carry this particular piece of baggage. Our patients bring this same piece of baggage into the clinical encounter. Our patients feel entitled to our care. It does not matter if they have no money or social stature and are on Medicaid, or if they have all the money and social stature in the world with Big Blue in their wallet; their feeling is that "it is free for me and I deserve your care." More than deserving it, they DEMAND our care.

While we may be going through the motions, providing goods and services, giving them the cure, they still want True Care, and they actually get angry that we are not freely giving our benevolent thoughts and emotions, our empathetic connection or compassion to them. When this is the case, they often act out and they get so angry that they mistreat us while demanding our care. They threaten us, tell us they are going to get us in trouble by calling administration, contacting the local paper, radio or television station. They even tell us it's our job to care; we have to care. Those situations never turn out well, for the patient or for us. Remember the patient who tried to kill me with his bare hands because he felt I did not care?

Here is a real story from a recent Medscape poll about "compassion fatigue" in emergency physicians. The sort of resentment and smoldering anger on display here is felt in hospitals all across the nation today. As you read about this patient encounter, remember, **it is not the patient's sense of entitlement that makes the encounter difficult; it is our reaction to that entitlement**. It is our inner feelings of anger, resentment or frustration that lead us to react rather than respond and keep us from connecting with our own desire to care.

> *A 23-year-old female presented to the ED via ambulance with an initial complaint of chest pain. When EMS arrived she gave a history of sub-sternal chest pain radiating to the left arm. She told EMS that she was allergic to nitroglycerin and morphine. Upon arrival to the ED the patient denied experiencing chest pain and then stated that her "real" complaint was a toothache x 1.5 months . . . and she wanted a refill on her Percocet. She had already seen a dentist 2 weeks ago. Her dentist had referred her to an oral surgeon for wisdom tooth extraction. The patient never made an appointment to see the oral surgeon. When asked why she called the ambulance for a toothache that had been present for 1.5 months she said, "I can call the ambulance anytime I want; my Medicaid will pay for it."*
>
> *Instead of treating this patient kindly and quickly, the normally mild-mannered ER doc exploded and began screaming at the patient, lecturing her on the proper use of the EMS/911, and how the ER was already*

swamped with emergencies and a "f**king" toothache for 1.5 months was definitely not a life-threatening emergency.

The patient began to cry. The patient called her family members and the hospital administrator. Several family members arrived at the ED and total chaos ensued with threats of violence by the family toward the ER doc, and reciprocating threats of violence by the 110 lb, 5 ft 1 inch female ER doc towards the patient and family. The hospital administrator, police department and the ED medical director arrived and wanted the ED staff to do whatever possible to please the patient to avoid the negative press.

Finally the ER doc gave the patient a prescription for Tylenol and Amoxicillin and discharged the patient.

Do you think this doctor felt good at the end of this patient encounter? Did this doctor create satisfaction for herself and her patient? Was this physician the cause of a new and better reality for herself and her patient? Or was she the effect of her patient, a broken system and a broken society?

What this physician reacted to, rather than choosing to take the time to respond to, was the patient's sense of entitlement. And she reacted out of her own sense of entitlement. This doctor, like many of us, feels that the emergency department is for real emergencies. Whether she realizes it or not, she feels entitled to take care of only "real emergencies." Toothaches are beneath her. She feels entitled to be treated as special, just because she is an emergency physician. She feels entitled to respect. She feels that the EMS System deserves respect, that it should be held in reserve for true emergencies. What if that ambulance was needed for someone who was really having a heart attack? And she is right, but being right in that encounter got her absolutely nowhere. Being sure you're right is a pretty sure sign that you won't be able to get yourself to that quantum space where satisfaction is found.

When it comes to searching for the problem in the quantum reality, where the problem is never the problem, typically the negativity you see in the one in front of you is inside you too. The reason the doctor was mad was because her patient felt entitled to get care from anyone in anyway she could. The doctor was mad because *she* felt entitled to deal with only "real" emergencies. We react when we see something negative in another that mirrors something in us we don't want to acknowledge. We react to seeing what we don't want to see. Understanding this can be incredibly helpful in real time when you're using the **TIME OUT** tool because it helps you to see the thoughts and emotions inside you that stand between you and your original, pure, uncorrupted desire to care.

All the patient did was push the doctor's button, her entitlement button. And all this doctor created for herself and her patient by reacting to the push of her entitlement button was pain, suffering, chaos and shame. This is what happens when we react rather than respond. This is the reality where we are the effect, not the cause. And this is our present reality.

The question we must all ask ourselves today, when the patient's behavior is challenging, is how can we effectively deal with this? It's not just entitlement—there are all sorts of reasons in today's society why our patients challenge us as caregivers. For example, with an aging population that's becoming demented, some patients can't actually remember what we just said to them. Likewise, it is very difficult to deal with mentally handicapped and mentally challenged children. Their behaviors are always challenging . . . and they can't help it. It is very difficult to deal with that.

This is something that plagues all of us, no matter who we are. We live in a society that is broken. People's dreams are broken and shattered, they turn to alcohol, they turn to drugs, and sometimes they have breakdowns. But they are still here, among us, and we want to care for them, we want to help them, because we know it is just the right thing to do.

But knowing this doesn't always make it any easier. When you are confronted with one of these situations, you have to remember that that person in front of you did not get up in the morning and look in the mirror and say, "I am going to do less than I am capable of today." **This is their best in the moment,** and though it's unimaginable to you that you could find yourself in such a situation, this is all they have to offer. **It does not matter if they are alcoholic, on drugs, demented, psychotic, or mentally handicapped: no matter what it is that renders them incapacitated, they are doing their very best.** And you can rest assured that you would not be standing in front of them if you did not have the desire and the capacity to care for them in some way.

In these situations, it is up to you, because you are the one in the equation who made the conscious choice to be here. It is not up to them. They were not born with a desire to put themselves in a condition to need your care. They need your care because they are overwhelmed by life itself. At some level of your shared humanity, there has to be a place where you can connect with them—even if it's the place of your own pain, where you yourself are struggling to care. It is up to you to dig deep and find that place within you, that quantum space, that will allow you to reach out and touch them with your humanity and feel their pain as if it were your own. **Could you imagine being in that situation, could you imagine not having the faculties to manage your life?** This question is your doorway into the empathetic connection that will allow you to turn on your own compassion for them. If you can reach that place, and touch them from there, you will find a word or an action that will allow you to express care for them and treat them with human dignity.

Often times in our families or in the hospital, in our roles as caregivers, doctors, nurses, medics, techs or even housekeepers, it seems as if those we are here to help are mistreating us. Deliberately going out of their way to make things difficult for us. It is at these times that we feel our righteous indignation, our automatic reaction, our automatic thoughts and feelings of *It's wrong, it's not fair* swell up from deep inside.

Under these conditions, caring for them can be the most difficult thing in the world to do. In moments like this, what helps us is remembering that the cure for compassion fatigue is to care anyway. What's more, **we have to remember that, in this** moment, "they" can't help it. **This is their best, and it is in our best interest to find a way to care for them anyway,** because as caregivers we chose to care, and the only way we can feel satisfied at the end of the day is do the difficult work, the extraordinary physical, emotional and spiritual work, that will bring about the extraordinary and the miraculous in our world. This is the synthesis of all the great spiritual wisdoms: love your neighbor as yourself.

How could this understanding, and the process I'm sharing with you in this book, have helped that poor, unfortunate, frustrated, weary emergency physician save the day in spite of her frustration? We can pretty easily see the steps she didn't take. First of all, she forgot why she came here: because she wants to care and make someone feel better. Second, she failed to realize that feeling good is up to her, and that in order to feel good she has to care. Third, she did not realize that she needed to recalculate the transaction with that challenging patient and find a way to give True Care anyway.

If our physician had had our framework and formulas, she would have known that once she had gotten through steps 1, 2 and 3, **Remember**, **Earn**, and **Formulate**, she could have moved on to step 4 and taken a **Look** at her position using the **TIME OUT** tool. She would have seen that it was her reaction to this patient's extreme sense of entitlement that stood in her way, and then she could have replaced those automatic negative thoughts and emotions with new thoughts and emotions, entering a new quantum space where she could give her True Care to her patient in a way her patient could receive.

For example, she might have told her patient how very sorry she was that she had to go through this experience of lying to 911 because she did not know any other way to get to the hospital. She could have given her a couple of pain pills to ease her pain now that she was here. Then our physician could have explained to the patient that her condition was not actually an emergency and that she was going to ask her to have a seat in the lobby or waiting area, because there were many patients here with true emergencies who needed the bed space more than she did.

Going further, our physician could have empowered her patient to do better for herself in the future. She could have shown her how making the effort to arrange follow up with the oral surgeon would actually have avoided this whole situation. The patient would not have had to suffer so long; she could already have been on the way to recovery. Our physician could even have offered to have one of the social workers help the patient make the calls she needed to make while she was in the waiting area, waiting for a bed space to open up in the emergency department.

It would have been a lot harder for the patient to be angry about this approach. Her pain and her situation would have been addressed. If the doctor had used our framework, her patient would be empowered to do better, not just given another prescription for antibiotics and pain pills and sent away until the next time. Both of them would have felt better, on both sides of the stethoscope.

Digging Deep

Simply knowing what we now know about the difference between cure and care, knowing how the quantum energies of care are subject to the laws of quantum mechanics, affords us the opportunity to undertake the difficult work of uncovering the negative thoughts and emotions that stand in the way of our caring. This is our only way out of our present situation. We must dig deep to find what is buried within each and every one of us. We must do the hard and unseen work of dismantling our own negativities and limiting beliefs.

When we hide behind our masks of self-righteousness, when we are unaware of what it is that makes us feel this way, we will find it impossible to be caring, even when we say we want to care. When we can finally get clear of these negative quantum spaces that stop us from caring, when we remove ourselves from these places, our caring will flow naturally, because humans are hard-wired to care!

While it won't be easy for us to see our own negativities, as they are buried deep in our unconscious memories and limbic system, if we are ultimately going to feel good, we must dig deep to find those negative thoughts, emotions and character traits, the flaws that we share with each other, and expose them. Once exposed, our collective negativities will be easy to overcome and dismantle. We need to uncover the constructs that limit us in the quantum world of thought and emotion, those thoughts and feelings that we are ashamed to admit, like the ones that stopped me from going to see a therapist when my patient passed away after he tried to choke me.

When we can see these things clearly, expose them, and name them, we will see just how limiting and useless they are. They will finally melt away and we will be free to care. We will be able to care without conditions. When we finally get to the place where we can love ourselves despite our flaws, our imperfections and our limitations, we will be able to see those hurting humans in front of us who want us to care, and we will be able to care for them despite *their* flaws, imperfections and limitations. We will be able to give our care unconditionally. We will have removed those things within us that cause us to judge or prejudge others as unworthy of our care. We will finally be clear to care.

Our personal and collective inner transformation is what enables us to be the cause, rather than the effect. This inner transformation is what allows us to put our own issues and baggage down long enough for us to clearly see why we came here, to see we want to help, to act as the cause of our patient's feeling better. From this place where we are clear about what we really want, we can inject thoughts and emotions into the patient encounter that will influence the thoughts and emotions of our patient.

With that in mind, in the next chapter we'll explore further how that inner transformation takes place and how to use the **TIME OUT** tool successfully when we meet our patient face to face in the quantum world.

Chapter 7

Look Out, Then Look In

Our experience of life is made up of the thoughts and feelings that we are experiencing at any given moment. These thoughts and feelings, whether we are conscious of them or not, shape our personal internal quantum space. Because of these thoughts and feelings, most of the time we do not feel good at work. We are on this journey for one reason and one reason alone: to find the way to a new internal quantum space where we do feel good at work. We are almost there; we are about to arrive at that feel-good quantum space where we can give care effectively in order to feel good ourselves.

We have a foolproof framework: when we **R.E.F.L.E.C.T.**, we guarantee our own success and generate our own personal and professional satisfaction. Let's review the steps in our framework so far:

1. **REMEMBER** what you came here for. Reconnect to your desire to care, to make a difference, to make patients feel better, to be the cause of your patient's feeling better because of your effort to care.

2. **EARN** your own satisfaction. You now understand that you are responsible for creating your own satisfaction, and if you are going to feel good, you have to shift your focus from the physical components of cure to the intangible energies of care.

3. **FORMULATE** your plan. You have learned how to recalculate the transaction of care according to the Perfect Equation, by which your giving True Care and your patient's receiving True Care add up to the energy of satisfaction in the quantum world of thought and emotion.

4. **LOOK** at your position within the transaction of care. Reframe your role in the patient encounter and your position in regards to your goal; ask yourself, are you the cause or the effect?

In the last chapter, you discovered that the obstacles to your satisfaction aren't outside you, but *within* you. Now you're ready to move more deeply into step four—to reframe your position in your personal, internal quantum space and complete the inner transformation of your personal neurochemistry that will move you from a negative space to a positive one, where you can give True Care freely and effectively.

Inner Space, Your Final Frontier

We now know about the difference between the physical tangible goods and services of cure and the quantum, intangible energies of thought and emotion that are the components of care. Giving care means we give our patient our benevolent thoughts and emotions while in connection with them. This is what allows us to feel good at work. The reason we do not always feel good at work is that something stops this from happening.

When something happens in our environment it triggers an automatic physiologic reaction in us that moves us internally into a negative space, a negative quantum space. In this negative space, we are completely disconnected from our desire to care. When we find ourselves in this internal negative quantum space, we need to use the **TIME OUT** tool and stop our instinctive reaction so that we can interrupt the automatic action-reaction cycle and, in that split second, choose to respond by injecting new positive thoughts and emotions instead.

To be able to use the **TIME OUT** tool effectively, we have to work to uncover our negative thoughts and emotions that construct the negative internal quantum spaces we find ourselves in. This work will be difficult. Why? Because none of us want to look at the baggage and garbage we carry around with us from all the times we've been hurt in encounters with others. This personal garbage is what builds our automatic defense mechanisms, designed by our unconscious or subconscious to protect us from being hurt again. Our amygdala and our limbic system's primary responsibility is to keep us from being hurt again. Think of them as a danger detector, and understand that in our role as care givers, this part of our physiology actually runs just beneath the surface of our consciousness and works against us—automatically and subconsciously.

I am asking you to look at your past hurts *while you are at work*— probably the time you feel least like probing your psyche. The reason I am asking you to do this is that our defense mechanisms really do not protect us. Instead, they cause us to act out in negative ways (like our emergency physician who was angry that a patient came to the hospital by ambulance for a toothache). Truth be told, our defense mechanisms actually lead us to make things worse for ourselves.

Let's face it, this looking at our baggage is not comfortable. It's not comfortable in a therapist's office and it is most definitely not comfortable when you are at work. It is uncomfortable looking at your own pain, just like it is uncomfortable to step into an encounter with another person in pain. Right now, I am asking you to tolerate your pain, just as I am asking you to feel and tolerate your patient's pain. In both cases I am asking you to tolerate pain without having a solution, without trying to fix that pain for yourself or for the patient. So in effect, I am asking you to feel uncomfortable as a means to an end, the end being feeling good at work, more and more often.

The **TIME OUT** tool is our doorway into our inner quantum space. We have to stop the automatic reaction of our unthinking beast within, our knee-jerk physiologic reaction, if we ever hope to be the cause of something better, something new and different. We are the cause of something better when we stop the cycle and inject our own benevolent, positive energies of thought and emotion into the system, into our patient and our environment. Why do we have to do this if we want to feel good? I'm so glad you asked.

Opening the Circuit

Ever try getting a flashlight to work when the batteries are in upside down? It won't work. There is a current and it flows in a specific direction. Energetic transactions between humans are the same: the energy flows in circuits just as electricity flows in any electrical device. Sound waves, X-rays, MRI waves, ultraviolet and infrared light rays, and even thoughts and emotions like hatred and compassion flow through circuits that carry energy in a certain direction and have a certain polarity to them.

When electricity flows through the circuit of a light bulb, it is converted to heat and light. When energy flows through the circuit formed by two people, it is converted to satisfaction. As long as energy is moving through this circuit, it creates a positive emotional state—it lights us up. When the interpersonal circuit of energy is interrupted, energy flow stops. When energy is not flowing, when the circuit is broken, the light goes out, and the result is a negative emotional state like anger, sadness or frustration.

I would like you to pay close attention now, because this concept is very important to your own emotional well-being, not just at work, but in life as well:

> **Happy, positive emotional states** are the result of a continuous flow of energy through the interpersonal circuit where the focus of consciousness is outward, on the other. We are happy when energy flows from us to another.

> **Sad, negative emotional states** are the result of stopping the flow of energy, when the interpersonal circuit is broken and the focus of consciousness is inward, on the self. We are unhappy when there is no

flow of energy between us and the other.

How can we use this information to improve our situation in the emergency department, in the healthcare system, and even in our personal lives? Let's look at it another way. Think of the difference between a closed pipe (a broken circuit) and an open pipe (a circuit that's working). How much water can you pour into a pipe that is capped on one end? Only a finite amount of water will fit in the closed pipe. When it is full, it is full; no more water can enter. How much water can you pour into an open pipe? An infinite amount: you can actually continuously pour more water into the system, because the water will move right through.

When it comes to being a caregiver, if your focus is on others and how you can help them and you are willing to invest energy in them and their situation, then you are acting like the open pipe and energy can flow through you to them. An infinite amount of energy can come into your system as long as you are giving it away to others. But the minute something happens to turn your attention away from the other, inward towards yourself—to make you think, *hey, what about me?*—the energy flow stops. You've capped the bottom of your pipe. You now care more about your own feelings and emotional state than about your patient's emotional condition. **This is why giving True Care**, **which creates satisfaction on both sides of the stethoscope**, **requires us to put our patient's needs in front of our own.** Remember the six-step process we must go through to create True Care described back in chapter four (Presence, Connection, Focus, Empathy, Compassion and Action)? We can't do this when we are trapped inside a negative quantum space where our focus is on protecting ourselves from being hurt, disrespected or mistreated.

In order to successfully care for our patient and create satisfaction for ourselves, we have to extricate ourselves from that internal negative quantum space—resentment, for example—and move to a positive space where we can once again make the empathetic connection and then feel compassion for our patient and genuinely want to give our positive thoughts and emotions to them, to be the cause of their and our feeling better. We must do this to be able to satisfy our primary, uncorrupted, pure and simple desire to care.

We must do this because **this is the only thing we can do to "feel good."**

Successful caregivers, the real heroes of healthcare, know that when we go outside ourselves and focus on helping others, there is no end to how much we can give, no end to the amount of compassion we can generate—and thus no end to how much satisfaction we can have for ourselves. The quantum effect of our giving is that now we can personally receive more.

It's when we stop giving that we stop getting—when we ask, *Hey, what about me? What about my lunch break? What about my lazy co-worker who is not pulling her weight? What about the fact that my boss does not appreciate what I do for these people? What about the fact that this patient does not respect me? What about the fact that the doctor thinks I am just his slave? What about the way this family is talking to me?* Me. Me. Me. When we are all inside ourselves, listening to the chatter in our heads, how they just expect us to take it, how arrogant and entitled they are, how stupid they are, how lazy they are, we only hurt ourselves. We break the circuit that is responsible for generating our satisfaction. We become broken circuits ourselves.

When you cap the bottom of your pipe, only a finite amount of energy can enter your own system. As you use that energy, you begin to feel drained. You have stopped the flow of energy in your system by turning the focus of your consciousness inward. You have closed yourself off, disconnected from your patient, disconnected from your environment. Without getting more energy to recharge you, you will feel sad and depleted. First you will feel dissatisfied and let down, and soon you will be depleted and burned out. If you keep your system capped and you stay focused on your own depletion, what you don't have, then you will start to augment and amplify your negative energies until they overflow in anger or lashing out at the other, which creates a mess in your environment.

Broken circuits pout, brood, feel sorry for themselves, throw temper tantrums and act out, just like our poor 110 lb, 5 ft 1 inch ER doctor who humiliated herself in front of everyone in the hospital, including the administrators and the directors of the emergency department. There is no satisfaction for us here in this place where energy does not flow. Unless we flip the polarity switch, open the pipe and allow the energy to flow again, we are doomed to have a negative work experience, a negative life experience.

In order to get the energy flowing again, we need to escape the negative quantum spaces that are generated by our automatic and inescapable physiologic reactions to people or situations in our environment. We need to move ourselves into positive internal quantum spaces where we can give our compassionate energies away.

How can we create these positive emotional states, especially when our environment challenges us so severely? How can we get back to a place of real engagement, happiness and joy, without sadness, depression, fears, jealousy or anger? The path we need to travel—the doorway into our power—is our care and concern for others. It all starts back at the beginning with remembering our pure, simple, raw desire to care and make a difference for others. This is where we find the strength to step outside our ordinary small selves, engage our compassion and become concerned with others' welfare, even when it seems they are (or they actually are) mistreating us, even when it is so very difficult. Our care and compassion for others allows us to move into a space where we can see that even though these people are behaving badly, they are doing the best they have the capacity to do right now. Here we can see that it isn't personal, it is not about us, and we can drop our judgments and concern ourselves with the burdens, worries and needs of these unfortunate ones.

In order to live extraordinary lives, we need to find the strength to stay outside ourselves. When we do, we become a channel for energy. This is when we create joy and happiness for our selves and others. This is how we change the world! This is how we activate the healthcare hero already within us and begin to enjoy the real, lasting, significant and meaningful stuff of life. The "more" to life I vowed I would find and have if God allowed me to survive cancer. Here it is, folks. This is it.

We have no choice but to step outside of our *Hey, what about me* mentality. Enough about me . . . **what about you?** What have I done for you lately? What can I do for you now? I want to apply this to everyone I come into contact with, but especially my patients, my staff, and my partners in healthcare. I know my happiness and my joy depend on flipping this switch.

The Quantum Merge

Never forget, doctors and nurses are people too! We are vulnerable to trauma and illness just like our patients. Any one of us could be involved in a terrible car accident or suffer a heart attack or stroke. Herein lies the key to unlock the door to that tender, honest, compassionate and empathetic place where we can touch our patient's lives and really make a difference. In order to establish a therapeutic relationship, we must make a personal connection. Making this connection is stage two in the process we go through to generate True Care.

If you have children, you probably have already experienced what it is like to really want the best for another, no matter how they have hurt themselves with the choices they've made. Unconditional concern and compassion is what we must tap into with our patients who have yet to find a way to quit smoking, lose weight, stop drinking, eat right, take their insulin, remember their blood pressure medicine or give up drugs. We have to look past the obvious problem to see the hurting human underneath it: the man who can't get out of the bottle of booze because he lost the love of his life to cancer.

When we see someone else hurting, True Care requires us to find a way to make our personal connection and then go deep into that connection to let the patient see we understand. It is our empathetic connection with our patient that allows our internal quantum space to merge with his or hers. When these two spaces merge, both parties know it, and change is created. It is in the moment when we establish that intangible energetic connection with the other that healing can begin.

When we engage in True Care, even when a physical cure is impossible, the quantum connection holds out hope for healing of another kind. I once heard the story of a young oncologist who had a friend from college contact him because his son was dying of a rare form of cancer. The man was desperate and he thought that maybe, just maybe, his old friend could use his connections to pull off a miracle for his son. The oncologist contacted everyone and every institution to see if there was anything that could be done, but after days and weeks of research, he asked his friend to come to his office. He just had to tell his friend face to face that there was nothing that could be done to save his son.

The young doctor shook his friend's hand and said, "I am sorry, but there is absolutely nothing that has been shown to be effective with your son's particular type of cancer. There's nothing I can do." With that, his friend hung his head low and walked out of the office.

As he was walking to his car in the parking lot, the young doctor came running after him. The man's heart lifted as he thought that maybe, just maybe, he had come up with a solution. But the doctor just looked at him, hugged him and said, "There *is* one thing I can do. I can sit and cry with you."

This is the energy of True Care, and you can see that it does not have to do solely with the cure or the outcome. Care is not just about history gathering, physical exams, diagnostic tests, treatments or prescriptions, about figuring it out or fixing it. Care is not about scripted explanations of wait times, procedures or service excellence. It's about feeling another person's pain and then wanting things to be better for them, turning on our own compassion for them.

Dr. Martin H. Fischer lived and worked in medicine roughly a hundred years ago, and he cautioned his medical students to remember "the aches": the headache, the stomachache and the heartache. He asked his students not to rely on labs or X-rays to define or understand these aches. Today we have become distracted by even more technology and we fail to pay almost any attention to the heartache, this basic human form of suffering. Dr.

Fischer knew that this ache did not exist in the body, it existed inside the patient's heart and mind, that intangible quantum space. In order to change things for the patient, you had to pay attention to both the tangible and the intangible.

Who among us has not suffered heartache and desperately sought relief? We can ache with desire for freedom from pain, freedom from suffering, freedom from worry, freedom from grief, and the only way to get any freedom is to feel that someone understands. Who could possibly understand better than your doctor or your nurse?

Patients come to us for true, authentic, genuine care, but make no mistake: the ability to care has nothing to do with a cure. They are two separate things entirely. One is tangible and the other is not. One is concerned with outcome; the other is all about the process. Our patients intrinsically know that in order for us to cure them, we must first care for them.

In some way they must understand that we are feeling their pain as if it were our own. This is where we close the space between us. This is where our quantum spaces merge. It is in the process of establishing this moment of empathetic connection that we become givers of care and our patients actually get that we care. This is why we can't fake care. This is why smile schools don't work. This merge has to be authentic to be felt. Anything else is patronizing.

It is in the moment of surrendering to the process of care that both the giver and the receiver can perceive the unique human experience of care. This is the circuitry of modern medicine at its most open and flowing. This is the quantum energy of True Care, and it is what we are both looking for on either side of the stethoscope. This is satisfaction for both the caregiver and the patient. This is where we will find our passion for medicine again.

The Best Cup of Coffee Ever

Time for a coffee break! It's always a good idea to take a break when you start to feel overwhelmed. I have presented so much information here, especially in these last few chapters, that you may be starting to wonder, *How do I put this all together so that I can feel good at work? How can all this talk of intangible energies make any real difference in what I deal with every day?*

Well, did you get your coffee like I asked you to? How is it? Is it good? Is it great? Is it awesome? Is it the best cup of coffee you ever had? Mine is.

What? I've lost you. OK, so follow this. I absolutely love coffee. Coffee has saved my life many times over. I have been working the night shift, eight hours, ten hours, twelve hours, sometimes having to stay over thirteen or fourteen hours to finish with my patients. I live my life sleep-deprived most of the time. What's worse, I recently found out I have a sleep disorder called sleep apnea. So let me repeat, coffee has saved my life many times over.

I love coffee. I love the way it smells. I love its color, I love its texture and I absolutely love the way it sounds when I put the scoop into the grounds. But there is nothing I love better about the coffee than the taste. I truly appreciate a great cup of coffee. I like mine strong, made light with whole milk and one packet of stevia. I don't like it with cream and I don't use sugar. Once I have made the best pot of coffee ever, I create the best cup of coffee ever, fixed just the way I love it. And then I savor the experience.

Those of you who have worked with me know that I always bring Pete's Ground Coffee with me to work. One of the very first things I do when I get there is make the best pot of coffee ever—and I inject love into the process: my love for coffee and my love for my co-workers. Once the pot is brewed I emerge from the coffee room and announce proudly, "I just made the best pot of coffee— EVER!" Somebody usually asks, "Did you make it with LOVE?"

Seems silly, right? But guess what, my co-workers have come to anticipate my awesome coffee. Their faces light up when I make my announcement. And if I know a particular nurse or doctor is too tied up at the moment to come and get some, I fix a cup for them, just the way they like it, and I walk the extra mile to take it to them, because there is nothing better for me than seeing the pleasure on their face as they take their first sip, while at the same time giving a phone report to the nurse on the floor.

This injection of love and care into food is nothing new. It is why pickles only taste good at Grandma's house. It is why nobody makes rigatoni like your Aunt Evelyn, and why nobody's chicken soup heals you like your mother's when you are ill. You and I can use the exact recipe and ingredients as Aunt Evelyn and Mom, but our rigatoni and soup don't really taste the same. This is because we can't possibly inject the same uniquely personal, intangible, quantum qualities of love, care, appreciation and dedication to our pleasure as Aunt Evelyn or Mom. Mom and Aunt Evelyn are fully engaged with the process of preparing our favorites for us.

Injecting intangible energy into physical matter and situations is something human beings have been doing since the dawn of humanity—and it's an essential element of our strategy for taming the beast within.

To see what this means, we need to look more closely at what's going on in our minds—and literally in our brains—when we're fully engaged with an experience. And the easiest way I know to talk about our level of engagement with ourselves, our hopes, our desires, our dreams and our personal mission in life is to look at the way we behave in relationships.

Think about love. Don't think about that bad old boyfriend; think about what it feels like to *fall* in love. In the beginning of any relationship, you are crazy in LOVE with the other person! You are blinded by this love. You don't see any of his flaws. You do not see any of her defects. You do not see any red flags. The sun rises and sets in this person's eyes. You know this one is the one and nobody can tell you different.

Can't eat, can't sleep, you just want to be with the one you love 24/7, you can't bear to be apart. You are officially in LOVE. People can tell. You are different because of that LOVE. You are so into this person, so involved, so enthusiastic and optimistic about your future together. If someone asks you why, you don't know! It has nothing to do with reality. It is all happening inside you: in your thoughts and emotions, in your head and your heart. It is in your mind, and most of all it's in your brain. Your prefrontal cortex is just dripping and oozing dopamine.

You date, you can't wait, your heart is all aflutter, you are most definitely "cuckoo for Cocoa Puffs"! Then it happens! He takes you to dinner at the most amazing restaurant. There is a stretch limo and a strolling violinist. He takes you to a show, drinks, then dancing. Suddenly on the dance floor, the music stops and the spotlight is on the two of you. The band plays "your" song as he drops down on one knee and slips ten carats on your finger. You've made it the top of the mountain. You are overjoyed that someone finally loves you just because you're you. All these intense feelings are swirling around inside you. Your prefrontal cortex is on overload. Congratulations, you have realized your wildest, most precious dream, and dopamine is actually dripping onto the floor.

He takes you back to the Ritz and you spend the night together. It is the absolute best you have ever had. You see fireworks. You feel the earth move. Your prefrontal cortex is showering all of your pleasure centers with dopamine, dopamine, dopamine and even more dopamine! You feel completed. Your dopamine receptors are entirely saturated. WOW, WOW, BOW, WOW, WOW!

The morning comes; you nearly kill yourself when you trip over the wet towel he left on the bathroom floor. You look at the towel, you are happy to pick up the towel, he was in such a hurry, so excited to be with you, how sweet, how cute. Even the experience of picking up that wet towel is pleasurable, because you LOVE him just because he's him. Your thoughts are focused on him: how great he makes you feel. How much you love him. How cute he is. You are definitely not thinking about you. The energy flowing through your open pipe is all directed outward, towards him, and you feel great!

Soon you are married and the honeymoon is over, literally. Time marches on, you grow accustomed to each other, and your prefrontal cortex begins adapting and decreasing the number of dopamine receptors available. It's just the way the addict's cortex adapts to heroin or cocaine: the high is never as high as the first time. Each time the addict uses, he needs to use more and more drug to get the same high.

You wonder, will you ever experience as much satisfaction as you had the night he popped the question, that night at the Ritz? You begin to get distracted by the business of life, the intensity of the feeling of being in love has faded just enough, and one morning on your way to the bathroom you nearly kill yourself when you trip over the wet towel on the floor. This time you're not thinking how sweet, how cute. Instead, you are cursing like a sailor. Why?

Even though that wet towel situation is the same as it ever was, because in the beginning you were so blinded by your love that you didn't mention that it bothered you, now you take the towel on the floor as a personal affront. Your thoughts are no longer about how wonderful he is, and they are now focused inward, not outward: the pipe is capped, the polarity is reversed, and you are now thinking how you don't get sweet text messages anymore. How you have not been out to dinner in months. How he works late. How you can't even get him to take out the garbage.

You feel he is taking you for granted and he doesn't appreciate you. You judge him as lazy and you resent him. Suddenly, it's all about you: what you don't have, what you are not getting, your lack, your need, your void. You are not getting what you deserve. You are not getting what you are entitled to.

Guess what, it is *still* all happening inside you. Your beast within, your automatic limbic-system-driven physiologic reaction, is now in control, because your prefrontal cortex is not getting any more feel-good dopamine simply because he is him. Your system has down-regulated the number of receptor sites available for him. Even though nothing in your physical external reality has changed—he never has picked up his towel—now you allow your emotions about what he's not doing to generate your negative thoughts about him, the same him you fell in love with. Now you find yourself complaining at work, at home, to your mother-in-law, to your colleagues at the hospital about that damn towel. You have given all your power away; you have renounced your free will to choose your thoughts, to inject positive thoughts. You have unconsciously chosen to become a victim.

You feel victimized by him and your situation. Entitlement turns to confusion and your thinking becomes flawed. You incorrectly reason that if he cared, if he really cared about you, he would pick up his wet towel and that would mean that he appreciates you and he really does LOVE you. In the split second when the towel transforms from being a symbol that you are with the one you love to being a sign that he doesn't care about you, in that moment when logic takes over, it is GAME OVER. It is only a matter of time.

You've just created a no-win situation for yourself because you will never be able to feel his love for you in the towel on the floor like you did the first time you picked it up. The first time you were wired on dopamine and your automatic thoughts were of him and how happy he made you by loving you. There was no logic back then, but now your logic and thinking have caused you to lose your desire for his love alone, refocusing it instead on his demonstrating his love by picking up the dang towel. So if he picked up the towel, would that mean that he really loved you? Does that mean that his love wasn't real when he didn't pick it up the first time? Really? Seriously now, what does picking up the towel have to do with you loving him or him loving you, anyway? Absolutely nothing.

In effect, what you have done to yourself in this adaptive physiologic process is that you have pinned your personal happiness to another person's behavior. Congratulations, you have just entered the wonderful world of co-dependency, addiction, depression, pain and suffering. Now there is no way for you to create your satisfaction or happiness on your own, for yourself. Now you can only feel happy or satisfied if he performs a meaningless task and picks up the towel.

What can we learn from this? In the beginning of anything, whether it's falling in love, getting a new job or even a puppy, the physiology is automatic. However, staying in love, loving the job and the puppy, is a conscious process that requires our ongoing efforts to overcome the process of adaptation, which is also automatic.

What is the way back to a feel-good, dopamine-rich experience? How can we get ourselves back? In any relationship, romance, friendship or professional situation, there's one simple tool. APPRECIATION! Appreciation is a sensitive awareness. Appreciation is an expression of gratitude, approval or admiration. To appreciate is to realize the value and importance of something or someone. It is a universal truth of quantum mechanics that when we lose appreciation for something, it is as if we no longer have any desire for it. It no longer holds any value for us. We no longer invest any energy into it. And without our energetic investment, we will not be allowed to keep it.

Watch a small child with a new toy. Initially, she won't let go of it. Every time she sees it, touches it, holds it, her prefrontal cortex starts to drip with dopamine, just like it does when the addict injects heroin. Dopamine is responsible for all of those good feelings our beast within loves so much. She doesn't want to eat, doesn't want to sleep and will play with it for hours on end until she has finally had enough. And then, suddenly, it is gone. That special toy is nowhere to be found. Why? It is our animal nature, our beast within. The physiological process of dopamine-receptor-adaptation has occurred. That toy is no longer the object of her desire.

How is it that what once brought us such joy, the toy, the puppy, the boyfriend, the job, no longer holds any satisfaction at all? With everything in life, you get out of it what you put into it. Look at all the effort we put into dating, the wedding, the proposal, and the planning of the honeymoon. After the initial efforts, most of us stop trying and just think we are entitled to wedded bliss the minute we return home. Look at all the effort we put into our degrees, the boards, and stressing over our first job. Most of us stop trying; we no longer inject any energy into the situation after our first paycheck, but just feel entitled to job nirvana. The key to reigniting anything, whenever we are starting to feel tired and lose interest, is to go back to the beginning, to reconnect to our original desire—

to go back to recognize and appreciate why we started doing what we're doing in the first place.

You can think of the beast within as your spoiled inner child who has an incredibly short attention span. Adaptation of the dopamine receptors in the prefrontal cortex happens very quickly. Success and satisfaction in life come when we continually put effort or energy into maintaining or improving the relationship with our spouse, our children, our parents, our careers. Why do you think every pot of coffee I make is the best pot EVER? Because this energetic investment in the process of preparing the coffee actually *creates* more dopamine receptors in my prefrontal cortex and allows my beast within to enjoy the taste of the coffee more. Gawd, I love dopamine!

The only way we can fight the physiological process of adaptation is to continuously inject positive energy (more receptors for dopamine) into a situation, open up the bottom of the pipe and let the energy flow through us toward others. Make it about them and their happiness. That is how we get it all. The house and the home. The best cup of joe ever! This is how we create or earn real and lasting happiness, joy and quantum levels of satisfaction for ourselves, for those we love, for society and for the planet at large. It is so simple, actually, yet so hard to do. How do we keep the satisfaction flowing?

Taking Back Control

I promised you that we'd come back and pay another visit to Matthieu Ricard, whose MRI research has so much to tell us about the physiology of *kara*. Ricard is a Buddhist monk as well as a physicist, and he has had his brain scanned on multiple occasions while meditating on different emotions. In a scientific study looking for the brain state that reveals happiness, his scans indicated that he is the happiest man on the planet when he meditates on loving compassion. And therein lies the key to taking control of our beast within—our automatic physiologic reaction, our limbic system and our amygdala that makes it so hard to stay satisfied with the work we do.

As we noted in chapter 2, Ricard explains that empathy is a cognitive process, an ability that humans enjoy, thanks to our prefrontal cortex, to resonate with another human being. If someone comes into our environment with a great big giant smile, through the cognitive process of empathy we feel happy and begin smiling too. This empathetic cognitive process can be conscious or unconscious, it does not matter, the results are the same: the areas in the brain that indicate happiness all light up. If someone suffers and you empathetically resonate with his or her suffering, the opposite happens. The area of the brain that registers suffering is activated so that you experience the suffering as well. Your experience is real suffering, and if day after day you suffer with your patients it can be overwhelming. It can make you burn out. As we've seen, the traditional method for dealing with this has been to distance ourselves: Don't get too friendly, set boundaries, be professional and stay clinical. We're taught that connecting with our patients' pain will engulf us, consume us and destroy us. But this is just not true. All the searching I have done shows us that it is not getting close that hurts us, it is not getting close enough.

The empathetic connection is part of Father Henri Nouwen's process for care, another stage in our process for generating and delivering True Care. This stage is required for our paradigm to work. It is the part of the reframing process that I call the Sinatra moment. Frank Sinatra was a genius! He sang *Do be do be do*, and in this case there is nothing to do; it's just a matter of *being* in empathetic connection. Staying in your patient's pain, not offering to fix it, not *doing* anything, just being with them in their pain until they understand you're feeling it with them, is what enables the shift and allows the energies of True Care to make a difference for them and for you. This is what we were describing when we spoke of the quantum merge. It is our empathetic connection with our patient that allows our internal quantum space to merge with his or hers. When these two spaces merge, both parties know it, and change is created. Then we can move into compassion and do or say something that will make all the difference in the world.

The amount of time you need to spend in this uncomfortable place of empathetic connection varies from patient to patient, according to the situation, but it is actually quite brief. Our fear of the pain is what stops us from entering into it, but once we find the courage to enter the pain, the fear is gone, as we clearly see that the pain does not destroy us; and when we take the next step and turn on our compassion, this enlivens us and actually empowers us. Entering the pain, our own or another's, gives us the power to move forward and inject the energies of compassion, loving kindness and human dignity.

Once we are in this state of compassion, the suffering areas in our brain are quickly deactivated and the areas of the brain that register wholesome, positive emotions like happiness and satisfaction are activated intensely. In that cascade that Ricard describes, dopamine begins to drench the prefrontal cortex of our brains. This is why caring for others, making a difference for others, feels so good to those of us who are born with the innate desire to care and make a difference. There is truly no better feeling in the world.

This is why I keep telling you, humans are hard-wired to care. When we don't act on this care, when we stay in empathy without moving deeper into compassion, we are hurting ourselves. When we get stuck in stand-alone empathy, when we are not connected to our patients, when we do not consciously move out of the state of empathy, we develop empathetic overload, a.k.a. compassion fatigue, which over time leads us to lose our humanity to the secondary PTSD of professional burnout. This is how we are hurting ourselves. There is a better way. When we effectively deliver real, authentic True Care to another, we get high, literally, on life. We feel good. We are personally healed from compassion fatigue and burnout. This is why we have to act on our pure desire to care. In this process, our efforts in the quantum space, working with intangible energies, effect a change in the physical matter of **our** brains, which feels great. This is quantum satisfaction. This is our end game.

When dopamine does not begin to flow automatically like it does inside the emergency—or the very first stages of being in love— we have to do the work in the quantum world and use our thoughts to make the dopamine flow again. We have an endless supply of dopamine in our bodies and we can be happy and satisfied all the time. It is when we expect to be happy for no reason, happy without doing our quantum work, that we screw ourselves into the negative emotional states of depression, sadness and anger.

The problem we have in modern medicine is that our fear of allowing us to feel the pain keeps us from entering that pain. Yet, avoiding pain always leads to more pain—in our case, compassion fatigue and ultimately burnout. Entering into the pain is the only mechanism that will allow us to finally feel good. We are talking about retraining our automatic reactive physiologic system, our beast within. They can train animals in the circus to face and enter into almost any fear. Circus animals will walk through fire as long as they know what the reward is that is waiting for them other the other side.

Consider this: why do we stay with a patient who is dying? It's painful to do this. But we know that we won't be able to live with our pain of knowing that she died alone. That pain will be worse the pain of staying with her until she takes her final breath. I came to fully understand this when my mother passed away. Embracing compassion is the only path to joy and happiness. Feeling another's pain feels bad, there is no denying this, but it's only stand-alone empathy that leads us to burn out. By moving into the state of compassion and injecting the energies of True Care, we be set free from dissatisfaction and burnout in health care—free to experience the best feelings ever.

Choosing to inject appreciation into our relationship inside the hospital and in our personal lives activates the dopamine and other neurochemical transmitters that help to keep us fresh, vibrant, dynamic and alive. Injecting our love and care into the soup gives it healing powers. Injecting appreciation and love into the coffee saves lives. Why do anything if you are not going to do it better this time than last time? What is the point unless the experience will be better, the high will be higher and the satisfaction will be greater? Will your next pot of coffee really be the best ever? Will your next encounter with a patient at work really be the best ever?

I told you that I would teach you how to create feel-good moments at work, and that with practice and effort, you could become so accomplished at creating these feel-good moments that you could quite possibly feel good most, if not all, of the time. In order to turn things around whenever we are challenged, frustrated or feeling badly, we can always take the option to use the **TIME OUT** tool and stop, turn our attention away from the trigger in our environment and turn our attention inward. We must focus on the automatic emotive process going on within us as a result of the action-reaction cycle found in interpersonal encounters.

We must see the thought constructs we are encountering internally, in our personal quantum space(s), and observe our thought stream with clarity. This is what the **TIME OUT** tool is for. This is where we can take control of our situation, where we can cause our situation to be better. This is where we can inject new thoughts and new emotions to change our personal internal quantum space. These new positive thought constructs will change the chemistry in our brain and allow us to experience something different, something better, something that actually feels good.

When I talk about taming the beast within, I am talking about our brain physiology, our brain chemistry, our dopamine, our serotonin and all of our neurotransmitters. It is now possible to see on MRI that just a thought can control them all, just the way we can discover that Matthieu Ricard is the happiest man on the planet when he meditates on unconditional love. We can see right before our eyes what happens on a MRI scan of the brain when we inject the thought (energy) of love, compassion and human dignity into our brains (physical matter). All the feel-good happiness centers in our prefrontal cortex light up, producing all sorts of endorphin-like chemicals that bathe our brains in feel-good juice. No wonder we crave this. How lucky for us that we have a built-in desire to care.

It turns out the Dalai Lama was right when he said, "If you want to be happy, practice compassion. If you want others to be happy, practice compassion." Effective compassion says I feel for you. Cognitive compassion says I understand you. Motivational compassion says I want to help you. Compassion is what allows us to engage with True Care and deliver True Care.

Compassion is the common denominator of all humanity. Our concern for ourselves is what separates us. Our concern for each other is what joins us. Imagine how much happiness or satisfaction you could create for yourself if your first thought about every person you encounter at work (or in life) was *I want to make it better for you. I want to care for you.* What do you think would happen? What if we could create a culture in modern healthcare where all of us were thinking all the time, *How can I make it better for you?*

As a group, in healthcare today, at the patient's bedside, we have a problem; we are letting our neurochemistry, our neurotransmitters, control us. It is clear with today's marvelous technology, designed to deliver cure, with the sophisticated and eloquent lesson the MRI scanner holds for all of us, that the solution is in gaining control our thoughts. Going through the discomfort of establishing and holding an empathetic connection with our patient and then identifying our reactive thoughts and emotions inside our personal quantum space and choosing to inject new thoughts and emotions that match our desire to give True Care—making it all about our patient's fears, needs and concerns, injecting unconditional love and human dignity to practice compassion—I feel for you, I understand you and I want to help you—well, this changes everything. This changes the world. This is what gives *you* the power to change the world and save the day!

Chapter 8

Recognizing Your Power

Once upon a time in the land of not enough satisfaction at work, we were unconscious of our own consciousness. We were unaware that satisfaction in general, and job satisfaction in particular, existed inside our personal and collective worlds of thought and emotion. Now we have explored our thoughts and emotions and learned more about them. We have journeyed inside our quantum world of human consciousness.

We used to think we needed things to be different at work in order to feel job satisfaction. We thought we needed circumstances to be different. We thought we needed superiors to be different or behave differently. We thought we needed co-workers to be different. We thought we needed patients and their family members to be different. We thought we needed humanity in general to be different. Now we know that this could not be further from the truth.

That ME, ME, ME, hey-what-about-me mentality is actually the cause of all of our pain and grief. We choose to be victims of other people, victims of circumstance, victims of the hospital, victims of the system, victims of the government, victims of the insurance companies, victims of the malpractice lawyers, victims of the patients. When we blame others for our dissatisfaction, we are clearly saying we are not responsible for creating our own satisfaction. This is a bitter pill to swallow. Just like in the movie

The Matrix—do you want to take the blue pill or the red pill?

The blue pill, well, nothing changes. You remain who you are today. Life is unfair. You don't matter. It's your lot in life to suffer. People are cruel. People take advantage of you. You get to go on blaming others for your shortcomings and inabilities. The End.

The red pill, well, everything changes. Your vision is transformed: you now see that all those things that you felt were holding you back, those things that are less than ideal at work and in life, those things are not what you want. Your new vision allows you to see the truth: chasing those things will always lead to frustration and disappointment. Life, your life, will never be the same; you can never go back. New life begins when you embrace the **TIME OUT** tool to find a way to give True Care, to put the needs of the other in front of your own.

Once you have swallowed that bitter red pill, in your new life you realize that you can never blame others for what you don't have, for not having what you want, and you realize that you can no longer complain; it is now against the rules. *Blame* and *complain* are both me-centered behaviors, and engaging in them will only bring us and those around us down.

Using the **TIME OUT** tool to reframe our situation is what will help us to come back from burnout and become the new heroes in healthcare. By suspending time for a split second, we create an opening to reconnect to our initial pure desire to help, and we inject new positive thoughts and emotions to change the personal internal quantum space we are in. When we act or speak from this shifted reality, we can change the world.

Let's review the steps we've gone through so far on this journey together:

1. Now you **REMEMBER** what you came here for in the first place, and you've reconnected to your desire to care, to make a difference, to make patients feel better *because* you care.

2. You've realized that you are responsible for creating your own satisfaction, and if you are going to feel good, you have to shift your focus from the physical components of cure to the intangible energies of care. You know that only you can **EARN** your satisfaction for yourself.

3. You have learned to **FORMULATE** your plan for getting the satisfaction that comes from caring, the good feeling that you crave. You have recalculated the transaction of care according to the Perfect Equation, by which your giving True Care and your patient's receiving your True Care add up to the energy of satisfaction in the quantum world of thought and emotion. You have learned to free yourself from your (hidden) agenda.

4. You now understand how to **LOOK** at your position within the transaction of care and ask yourself if you are the cause of something better or the effect of another's situation. You now ask yourself, am I reacting or am I responding? You know how to reframe your role in the patient encounter and your position in regards to your goal: you understand that the obstacles to your satisfaction aren't outside you, but within you. You know how to make the inner transformation and shift your position in your personal, internal quantum space from a negative to a positive one.

5. Now you're ready to take step 5, where you'll learn to **EVALUATE** your thoughts and behaviors and recognize whether or not they are helping you to be successful. You will understand how to use your own power to create satisfaction for yourself, your co-workers and your patients.

Once you have reframed your position and used the **TIME OUT** tool to inject new positive thoughts and emotion into your energetic caring system, you have delivered True Care and made a difference for your patient. By now, you can recognize what is happening as it's happening. You recognize when your patient relaxes, takes a deep breath, smiles, and feels better, because you've been successful at delivering True Care. You can also recognize that when you are feeling frustrated, your patient is frustrated, and neither of you is feeling satisfaction. You can recognize when you don't feel good. In short, you can recognize the power you hold to create your own experience—to create your world, moment by moment.

You exercise this power simply by the thoughts you choose. Inside your own world of thought and emotion, you and you alone have the choice; if the thoughts and emotions you are experiencing do not serve your emotional well-being, you can choose to replace them, to inject new thoughts that allow you to be the cause of your own satisfaction in any interpersonal encounter. With this choice, the thoughts you inject will be those that allow you to open up and give your care to another. When you choose to allow the quantum energies to flow through you, you will always create a positive emotional state for yourself; you will always feel happy and satisfied.

I Think, Therefore . . .

Our thoughts are powerful influencers of our experience. Perception is reality, or is it? There is way more here than meets the eye. How can two patients involved in the same car accident, house fire or trauma have such radically different stories? How can the patient who complains to your boss about you have such a different story than you do about what actually took place? Your perception of the situation is 180 degrees opposite to their perception. What gives? What exactly is reality?

We generally think of our reality as our perception of our experience. We perceive with our five senses. No two people perceive exactly alike, and therefore no two people experience anything in exactly the same way. There are tons of things going on in what we call "reality" that we are mostly unaware of. Things that we can't see, hear, smell, taste or touch. We all know germs are in our reality, but we can't perceive them; we don't have the sensory apparatus. This does not stop us from using universal precautions, donning gloves, gowns and masks, buying sanitizing hand creams and using Clorox wipes. We are conscious of the fact that germs exist in our reality, and we act on this information, even though we do not have the senses to perceive their presence. Our reality includes germs even though we can't perceive germs, unless we augment our five senses with a microscope.

Many of our patients, on the other hand, still do not understand about germs. They may feel certain that you get a cold just from being in the cold, or from being cold. It only follows, then, that they believe that they got cold from going outside without a jacket, or an earache from going outside without a hat. For these people to feel good, in their reality, they must wear a hat when they go outside in the cold. This becomes their experience of reality.

For many of us who work in healthcare, our reality includes X-rays, which are dangerous. We wear radiation sensors if we work in X-ray or fluoroscopy and we act on this knowledge of the danger of X-rays, even though we as human animals do not have the sensory apparatus to perceive them. The point is that **we bring what we know to be true into our experience of reality. In other words, we color or interpret the information our five senses are presenting our brain with to formulate our personal experience of reality.**

Although there are five human senses, sight, hearing, smell, taste and touch, not all of us have access to all five senses or access to the same quality of information from them. Each sense works differently, and each of us uses one sense preferentially. Some of us have to hear the information to learn it, some have to see it, and others of us have to feel it or learn experientially.

Take the sense of sight, for example. We literally see the world upside down. The optics involved actually project an image onto our retinas that is inverted. It is our brain that interprets right side up the information it receives from the retinal receptors, and our brain's interpretation of the information it receives then becomes our experience of sight. In other words, our experience of sight is not just raw information. Our experience of sight is actually an interpretation of our "reality."

Our four other sensory experiences are also our brain's interpretation of raw information coming through receptors in our nervous system. Our brain's interpretation of the sum total of the information coming from our physical body's sensory apparatus creates our perception of our physical reality. Yet our brain's interpretation of our sensory information, what we sometimes call our perception, is not yet our "experienced reality." **Our experience of reality is the sum of our perception(s), plus our thoughts and emotions, plus our memories at the time that sensory information is received. Our cognitive and emotional states color, tint, shade, shape and influence what we ultimately experience as our reality.**

Our perceived experience of reality, then, is our brain's interpretation of reality filtered through our thoughts, including our own personal past experiences, which hold our world view and operating system (even if your operating system is flawed because you believe that you get an earache from not wearing a hat) as well as our emotions in the moment. We are sentient beings, meaning that we have the power of perception by the five senses as well as the power of consciousness. Sentient beings combine systems of sensory information with those systems of cognitive information and emotional awareness.

Sentient beings' experience of reality thus combines the physical system (matter) and the energetic system, the quantum world of thoughts and emotions that we've been exploring in such depth. Our thoughts, our emotions, our beliefs, our past experiences are always shaping our brain's interpretation of our present reception of sensory data. How many times have you heard someone you love tell you that you see only what you want to see, hear only what you want to hear? Everyone around you somehow seemed to know that boyfriend was no good for you, but you saw none of his flaws at the time. How many times have you told a patient something about his diagnosis or his care and realized later that he did not hear a word you were saying? How many times has a patient asked you to write down what you are telling her so she can remember it, because she knows she is not thinking clearly right now, she's too emotional?

Our experience of reality is our perception plus our consciousness—so it should be blatantly obvious by now

that we have the power to change our reality by changing our consciousness. Our good or bad feelings depend on the thoughts we choose to engage, for our thoughts change the neurochemistry happening in our brain's experience center, the prefrontal cortex. This is where we mix the two systems, physical matter and the energetic spectrum. This is where our two worlds collide, the Newtonian world and Einstein's quantum reality.

In our framework, once you recognize that you are experiencing frustration or dissatisfaction, you can change your experience, and the experience of those around you, by changing your thoughts and emotions, by taking control of your consciousness. In order to do this you have to understand and be aware of the automatic autopilot action-reaction cycle, interrupt it and then inject new positive emotional and thought energy into the system to change your experience, as we've been discussing in the last two chapters. **You have always had the power to change your experience of reality; you now know how to control it.**

Setting the Bar Higher

Now that we know how we can create our own good thoughts and feelings when we are paying attention to what is happening in our own personal quantum space, becoming consciously aware of our automatic, autopilot reactions that come from our animal nature, our amygdala and our limbic system, it is time to take a closer look at what happens when we *aren't* paying attention. When we are not aware of our stream of consciousness, when we are on autopilot and automatically reacting to our environment, our unconscious, animal-like, automatic neurochemistry is in control. Let's look at the ways we let this behavior in us inhibit us from extracting joy, pleasure and satisfaction from our environment.

Our animal-like reactive nature is basically self-centered and self-serving in its desire for immediate gratification. When we are hungry, we eat to feel better. When we are angry, we lash out to feel better. But fulfilling our desire for immediate satisfaction plants the seeds of our long-term dissatisfaction. It's the primary reason we find ourselves smack dab in the middle of our broken dreams, broken systems, and broken society filled with broken individuals.

In healthcare, broken people and systems in collapse or decay surround us. It can seem like we live in a time of intense greed where the only thing anyone can concern himself or herself with is I, I, I.

We as caregivers are seen as special, different, sort of like clergy. Society recognizes that we signed up, made the conscious choice to provide care. We are seen as having special gifts and special talents. We are held to a higher standard than the people we care for. This double standard is part of the reason why we feel so helpless and overwhelmed. We often feel we cannot say what we want to say, what our patients need to hear. We dare not speak the truth. (*You can't breathe because you are obese.*) In the midst of this, many of us, as caregivers, feel hopeless. Thankfully, this very same double standard is what will help us to find the way out of this dark, angry place we find ourselves in now.

Ungrateful, entitled people are hollering at us all the time. They want instant gratification. They want instant diagnosis, instant treatment, they want instant relief and they want to feel our care— instantly. They want what they want and they want it NOW. They call the administrator when they don't get these things instantly! And here is where that double standard applies. It is never "OK" for us to react at our patients' level. What, then, are we to do with our own negative thoughts and emotions? We just have to look at the problem and then the solution will become obvious. What are we currently doing with our negative thoughts and emotions?

Most of us feel that things have deteriorated and we blame that deterioration on patient satisfaction surveys, political correctness, patient complaints, the government and the lawyers. We know that these things lie out of our control, so what do we actually do with our angst? We complain incessantly about being overwhelmed, overworked, underpaid, underappreciated, disrespected and overscrutinized. When complaining doesn't fix our problems, we turn our anger on each other. This has affected the way we all treat our staff, our co-workers and our peers. We are less supportive of each other. We are less kind to each other.

We act out our anger in subtle and less subtle ways, by complaining, trash talking, gossiping, judging, shaming, righteous indignation, controlling, passive-aggressive behaviors and entitlement issues. This acting out gives us some instant gratification, and temporarily eases our pain, but it ultimately creates even more dissatisfaction and depletion for us.

Some of us are saying, *I just don't know if I can do it anymore. I don't think I can tolerate the junk anymore, the BS. It is affecting the way I think of myself. It is affecting the way I think of others. It is affecting the way I think of society. It is affecting the way I treat others. It is affecting the way others treat me.* Some of us are asking, *How can I continue to care for people, please tell me! How can I stay in healthcare, how can I collect a pension? How can I work in this situation without more of those feelings that come from magic moments of helping others and saving lives?*

Did you notice something in all of the sentences above? The powerless feeling stems from the sense of being a victim at the mercy of all that is going on around you. If you are looking for the magic answer, you must recognize that you are responsible for creating the magic. You are responsible for creating your own satisfaction. Nobody can do it for you, nobody can fix it for you, and nobody can give it to you. You and you alone are responsible for your happiness. And from everything that I have told you so far, you must recognize that you will never make the magic, feel the satisfaction, create the fulfillment you are looking for, if you only concern yourself with what it is you are *not* getting. When you are thinking, *hey, what about me,* you can use the **TIME OUT** tool to snap out of it! Right now, in healthcare, in this moment of despair, you can recognize where you are stuck inside yourself and recognize the power you already have within you to turn it all around.

If you are looking for respect, give respect. If you are looking for appreciation, find things to appreciate. It will not be easy, and it will require you to continually transform internally by recognizing that the obstacles to your satisfaction are not in your environment, they are the reactions inside you. It will not be easy, but the rewards will be great.

Bad Behavior 101

We work in relationship to each other and our patients. In any relationship, if it is not good, it's bad. If it does not heal, it harms. If it does not join, it separates. Human dignity is the Golden Rule for feeling good. Treat others as you would want to be treated. Love your neighbor as yourself. Do not do unto others what you would find odious if done to yourself.

Almost all our bad behaviors exist because they temporarily alleviate our discomfort, usually at the expense of another. They are intrinsically selfish and they allow the "me, me, me" to feel good right now. Every bad behavior has a "me" focus. We have seen that this polarity caps the pipe and does not allow the flow of energy we need for our long-term satisfaction.

Acting out is what we do when we are not getting what we want; think of a two-year-old having a temper tantrum. Acting-out behaviors allow a short burst of intense energy that feels good for a second, but they are followed by bad feelings, guilt, shame and chaos. In the final analysis, they always cause us to feel drained and empty, depressed and depleted. They are much like electrical short circuits, when a light bulb burns out. This is what burnout is in our profession. This is why we feel we have to leave the profession. All acting-out behaviors are circuit breakers. They break the circuit of energy that we have to establish if we want to feel good at work.

Here is a romp through all of the negative behaviors we indulge in that leave us in a worse situation than before. Like eating a lot of chocolate, only to find out we have gained ten pounds later in the week. It felt good, but was it worth it? All of this is presented as a starting point so that you can recognize where you are stuck in your workday, so that you can use the **TIME OUT** tool to flip the switch and get about the business of creating more and more feel-good moments for yourself.

Complaining. No good will ever come of it. Whining, bitching or moaning focuses the energy of others on you for a minute and gives you a little boost, but ultimately it causes others to lose respect for you: in the end, no one will take you seriously. The sky is not falling. When you find yourself complaining, just stop. Then begin looking for something, anything, that is working or good around you. Make it a habit to focus your energy on looking for the good in any situation. Appreciation of any kind is the antidote to the energy drain of complaining.

Overwhelmed. The minute you say it, you are rendered powerless. Don't say it! If you are feeling overwhelmed, look for any small thing you can do for your patients or co-workers. Even a smile will start the positive energy flowing. Say thank you, ask, "What can I do for you?", pick up the wet towel on the floor. The smallest action will uncap the pipe and get the energy flowing through you again, energizing you and empowering you to do more than you thought you were capable of doing.

Avoidance. This is always a sign that we already know there is a problem. We just do not want to face it. Whenever you recognize that you are avoiding a person or situation, go, face it now, because each second that you avoid it, the problem will enlarge, augment and amplify itself. The energy drain of avoidance is always greater than the actual situation you are avoiding. SO GO NOW! Face the situation and make it about doing something for them. When you see a patient's family member standing outside the curtain giving you the evil eye, brooding, looking as if they think no one cares about them or the patient, don't turn away— face the situation. Ask, "Was there something that you needed? Something I can help you with?"

Judging. This is a way to feel instantly better about yourself for a whole two seconds. It is always easier to care when you haven't judged or deemed someone unworthy of your care. Who are we to judge anyway? When you find yourself judging someone, anyone, stop and look for a way to see past the distractions, beneath the bad behaviors and the sense of entitlement. Remember that patients weren't born with a desire to be in need; they are in that moment doing the best that they are capable of. Find a way to see that this one is hurting and needs to be treated with human dignity. Find a way to drop the judgments.

Passive-Aggressiveness. This behavior always stems from our judgment of another. Start looking at the thoughts behind your actions. When speaking with a patient, are you frustrated or angry with the person or the situation you are in? When you're asking, "How are you feeling?" are you really thinking, *What's wrong NOW?* Passive-aggressiveness creates "You don't deserve it and you can't make me give it to you" no-win situations. These almost always lead to the power struggle, the extreme situation where I will be polite but you still can't make me give it to you. Recognize that the energy behind your actions is creating your bad day. When you smile or say thank you, work on meaning it.

Manipulation. Although many of us are quite skilled at this, it never works in the long term. Manipulation is what humans do when they feel that straight-up asking for what they want won't work. Are you afraid to ask for help? Are you worried you won't get what you want or need? Begin transforming this behavior by looking for things you can do for others, especially those things you would like others to do for you.

Entitlement. This is always a death sentence as far as satisfaction is concerned. Anytime we feel that we deserve, we become stagnant, and then we're headed towards a dead end. The best way to avoid the entrapment of entitlement is to exchange the desire to be right in any given moment for your original desire to care for others. Remember, you are most likely right about all the things you deserve, but is it getting you anywhere? When you begin to feel you aren't getting what you deserve, recognize that you are stepping right into quicksand. Stop, refocus your attention on your desire to care, and inject this positive energy into your next action.

Shaming. We are all good at this. We do it anytime we embarrass someone or bring blood to their face. We may say to a patient, *You should have thought about that before you got hurt. You should have thought about that before you did the drug.* Take a look at who you are picking on, you big bully. Shaming is designed to make you feel better about yourself. Do you really need to feel better than the alcoholic or the drug addict? Most often, when we shame someone, it is because we've spoken in reaction to what we see in that person. It is not what you say, but the consciousness behind what you are saying, that is doing the harm. If you stop yourself from reacting and work to inject compassion and kindness into your words, your words will be transformed, not causing shame but creating awareness for the person you are speaking to.

Righteous Indignation happens anytime we feel the need to stop others from acting out with their bad behavior. It's also a surefire way to generate a patient complaint. Many times the behavior we seek to stop really does need to be curtailed, but how often are we successful when we act from indignation? When you feel the righteousness starting to rise up in you, stop, recognize your indignation and inject positivity into your consciousness before you act.

Gossip and Trash Talking are truly two of the very worst behaviors. They're essentially the same thing as shaming, except more damaging to you, because the person you are shaming is not even present. Gossip is very hard to resist, very seductive. Large amounts of negative energy result, and it creates huge, devastating, lasting damage to the fabric of a team. Trash talking, too, is something many of us are good at. We turn our angst and anger on each other, complaining that others are not seeing enough patients or pulling their fair share of the load. This breaks the circuit for long-term satisfaction because it creates separation, not unity. The damage is often irreparable, because once you say it you can never take it back. Imagine that negative words are salt and positive words are sugar. Get a saltshaker and a bowl of sugar. Take the salt and pour it into the sugar. Now remove the salt from the sugar. Impossible, right? The salt will always be in the sugar. There is a way, however, to fix the sugar. That is by adding even more sugar, eventually diluting the salt to the point where the sugar no longer tastes bitter, even though the salt is still there. So every time you feel you want to speak negatively about someone, stop yourself and find something sweet to say instead. If you can't find anything sweet, don't say anything at all.

Flipping the Switch

As you can see, all of the behaviors above can be switched into something positive. When you engage in the creative process of injecting positive thoughts and emotions into your present moment of feeling bad, you are investing your own energy in your environment, leaving your mark, making a difference, creating a new reality that feels much better. Use the **TIME OUT** tool to flip the polarity switch and soon you and everyone else will be feeling better, feeling good.

Yes, we are hurting. This truly is a painful place to be in. Focusing inward, holding the pain within us, makes us feel worse and, yes, we act out. We lash out at each other, because we can't lash out at the patient or our boss. Yes, for a brief second, we feel better, but ultimately things get worse. Yes, it would appear that we can't get no satisfaction.

But this could not be further from the truth. Now that we can recognize consciously where we are, we can see that this is nothing but illusion. We must fight our animal nature and tame our beast of neurotransmitters within. We can do this with the knowledge we now have about Einstein's quantum reality, the way energy and matter are intrinsically related and the laws that govern the energetic transactions between humans. We can use the **TIME OUT** tool to inject new thoughts and emotional energy into our consciousness that will allow us to rise above our animal nature and create feel-good satisfaction more and more often. The reward will be sweet and everlasting.

We came to this life and these jobs to give care. Every time we give and share, it makes us feel good because we connect to our true purpose and mission. In our present defining moment, we are facing challenges around giving. When we feel like we are doing a favor for others by giving to them, we need to recognize that we are creating short circuits in ourselves and our environment. When we are looking for appreciation and respect and we do not feel we are getting these things, our reactive behavior is to stop giving.

The question is, are we really doing anyone a favor when we give our care? We already know that the person who benefits the most from the act of giving is the giver. By opening the energetic circuits through our giving care to others, we will attract to ourselves and create for ourselves health, wealth, peace of mind, meaning and a sense of purpose, as well as happiness and satisfaction, on all levels of the quantum field. Knowing this, we should be chasing opportunities to give care. We must understand that if we really want to have all that this life has to offer, it does not matter if we are appreciated or loved because we are giving people. In the final analysis, all that really matters is that we are givers, period.

Our key to really caring is to really listen. We must listen with our heart and not our ears to what our patients are trying to say. What pain is there behind the words they are saying, the bad behaviors they are displaying? How much pain is there inside them that is covered with all those things they are trying to show as strength? To be able to hear their pain will allow us to care for these hurting humans, especially those of us in healthcare, because we are hard-wired to care. Sometimes, just listening, caring about their situation, is enough to manifest a change, to make them feel better.

Let me introduce you to a few of my friends who can help you do this in your own life and work, day in and day out. It my sound silly, but I could not be where I am today, happy and resilient, if I did not chant their names over and over again while at work. Meet Tolerance, Kindness, Compassion, Caring, Empathy, Sympathy, Giving, Sharing, Hope and Grace. Make them your friends too, and bring them with you to work and to the bedside. When you are tempted to judge another person, invite compassion to the bedside, because compassion knows that this is the patient's best. She did not get out of bed, look in the mirror and say to herself, *I am going to do less than I am capable of today*; this, in this moment, no matter how repulsive it seems, is her best.

Working in healthcare, we put a sign outside that in effect says, "Care inside." In fact, one of the hospitals where I work has a literal sign—a huge red-and-white sign above the entrance to the Emergency Department that boldly proclaims "EMERGENCY

CARE CENTER." We must always understand that we are the ones who come to this situation willingly, advertising that we are here to give care. But care is not a substance that can be pulled from the drawer in the Pyxis station. It's not something you can take down from a shelf. And it's not something that inherently exists inside the walls of the hospital building. The care people expect to find will come from the people who work there, the ones at the patient's bedside.

So we must care and show mercy through our kindness. We must move out of our resentment and step outside the ordinary. Our patients want to feel our merciful care for them so that they can briefly, if only for a moment, forget about the terrible situation that brought them to us in the first place. And we chose to be here so that we could have the opportunity to give it to them.

We couldn't get the satisfaction we seek from being caregivers without people who need us. No one wakes up with the desire to be needing us today, but we wake up every day with the desire to take care of others in need. Remind yourself of this every time you walk through the doors.

When we connect with our patients through empathy and then turn on the compassion and deliver care or love for no reason, we enter the energetic quantum space where we find the magic we are looking for. This space exists beyond time, space and motion. When we interrupt the automatic action-reaction cycle with the **TIME OUT** tool, it is as if time stands still and the space between caregiver and care receiver disappears.

When we connect with our pure and simple desire to help, it is always easy to help, if you can use the **TIME OUT** tool to step outside your automatic reactive behavior and not judge, eliminate the attachments to your giving care, drop the agenda and care just because you know caring will make you both feel better. To do this, think of yourself as a tourist. Think like a tourist. This concept will allow you to see through the entitlements, the arrogance and the bad behaviors, because tourists are only interested in seeing the good on their journey. Or think of the person in front of you as a car and look under the hood; see underneath his situation, his baggage and his disguise.

People really are your greatest tool when you see them as your mirror for the universe. You know that when you smile the whole world smiles back at you. When you are irritated or angered or feel that someone in front of you is pushing one of your buttons by the way they are treating you or talking to you, realize that you are really only irritated because you are seeing one of your own flaws or imperfections mirrored back to you. If you spot it in another, you got it; it's yours. It is easier to find compassion for another when you can find compassion for yourself.

You have just looked into that universal mirror and seen your own reactive beast within. It is time to tame that beast, control that animal nature of ours and become self-responsible. We must be 100 percent responsible for our own satisfaction, success and happiness. We can never lay blame on others for our own lack of satisfaction or fulfillment. We cannot complain. Not if we are truly self-responsible.

If we do not have what we want at work, or in life, we simply have not worked hard enough to create it. Life is what you make it. Recognize that if we don't have what we want from this life, we have not invested enough energy in the process—we simply have not done enough work to create it.

We are the lucky ones, we are the ones fighting the good fight, we are the ones fighting the beast within. No matter what your worldview or your personal persuasions, at the end of your life, when you go to meet your maker, and they ask, *What did you do with your life?*, you can say, *What I did was meaningful, what I did was powerful, what I did was important, what I did made a difference.* You can say I worked in the Emergency Department, I worked in healthcare, I was a medic, I was a health unit coordinator, I was the one who registered them, I mopped up the blood, I took out the trash, I was a nurse, a physician assistant, a manager, an administrator, a nurse practitioner, a doctor.

You can say, I was on the team! I did my best! I changed the world, one patient encounter at a time, and created satisfaction on both sides of the stethoscope.

Chapter 9

Back to the Beginning

The steps I have taken on my own healthcare hero's journey have brought me right back to the very beginning. That place in my parents' backyard in Pennsylvania where I was bandaging up all the stray dogs in the neighborhood, acting on my desire to care, to make it better. All of that play was going on in my imagination, in that prefrontal cortex where all those rich feel-good neurotransmitters reside.

These steps that I have taken on my journey have brought me right back to this place where I now realize that I've always had what I always wanted, a pure and uncorrupted desire to care. All the degrees, the training, the diplomas, the merit badges, all of the angst and reaching for the wrong things in my life and my career, have brought me home to the very same place I was fifty years ago—a place where I understand clearly that all I ever wanted was to care and be cared for.

While I struggled in my personal life, after beating cancer twice, to get the more that life had to offer, I was only struggling and not finding the answer. It was through my conscious journey, my quest into my dark night of the soul, that I realized I was happiest in my practice of medicine at the free clinic caring for patients without pharmaceuticals or treatments, when all I had to give was my care.

My true healing from cancer began when my surgeon wrapped his arms around me and held me as I cried. When he held me, he connected with me through his empathy, feeling my pain so that when he offered his compassion, we both felt better. He promised me that he would do everything in his power to make it better, and he did.

My first glimpse into my problem with satisfaction at work came when another physician stepped up to care for my patient because he cared for me. He gave me True Care by connecting to my frustration and empathizing with me, feeling my pain, and then compassionately offering to take my patient to the operating room to make it better for me.

Stepping into the emergency for Adam and his parents allowed me full access to all of my gifts and talents so I could bring all of them to his bedside to do what seemed impossible, to participate in a Lazarus moment. I, like everyone else involved, was automatically consumed with empathy for Adam and his parents and we acted together in compassion, activating True Care to make it better for all of them. Our limitations fell away as we naturally rose to the occasion.

And finally there was Joseph, the patient I did not feel care for, who ended up trying to kill me because he felt—he *knew*—I did not really care about him. I was his doctor, I was supposed to be the one who cared for him, and I let him down. This was the final blow to my old way of thinking, for the pain and the suffering, the angst and the despair that I felt as a result of Joseph's death, when no one, not even me, really cared for him, was more than I could bear.

Through all the experiences in my life and my career, it became clear to me that caring for others and being cared for by others were the situations where I felt the most alive, where I experienced the more that life has to offer. These were the places where all of the miraculous happened for me and for those around me. These were the enlightening steps that I took on my own healthcare hero's journey.

After I understood better the steps of my journey, I spent the next little while formulating the contents of this book and the framework

I have shared with you. As I worked on it, though, I was not always successful at creating quantum amounts of satisfaction for myself, and some days were even harder than others. Many of my old feelings started surfacing again, and I slipped back into my "hey, what about me" victim mentality. I had to do the hard work of applying the framework I have given to you here over and over again, transforming myself internally each time so that I could be the cause of a new and better day, more and more often.

There is an old saying that nobody cares what you have done; they only care about what you are doing. Well, our brains don't care what we have thought in the past; our brains only respond to what we are thinking right now. In order to inject positive thoughts and emotions into every situation, I had to work and work hard to overcome my animal-like reactive nature, my autopilot, my automatic physiology.

This is difficult to do even knowing what I know, especially when the patients are acting entitled and ungrateful, the staff is grumpy and irritable, and there seems to be no joy in Mudville. It is a huge undertaking to abandon your old reactive operating system and act from a new one, especially when you need to get things accomplished right now. Ever migrated from Windows XP to Vista, or Windows 7 to 8? Ever moved from Windows to a Mac? Even though I've researched and successfully used this new practice of causality and mind-over-matter technology, I still have to regroup and start again to apply it effectively: to remind myself of the process, the perspectives, and the insights and use the **TIME OUT** tool to carve out the inner space to care.

Let's see how this step fits into the framework we've been following all through this journey:

1. Now you **REMEMBER** what you came here for in the first place, and you've reconnected to your desire to care, to make a difference, to make patients feel better *because* you care.

2. You've realized that you are responsible for creating your own satisfaction, and if you are going to feel good, you have

to shift your focus from the physical components of cure to the intangible energies of care. You know that only you can **EARN** your satisfaction for yourself.

3. You have learned to **FORMULATE** your plan for getting the satisfaction you crave that comes from caring. You have recalculated the transaction of care according to the Perfect Equation, by which your giving True Care and your patient's receiving your True Care add up to the energy of satisfaction in the quantum world of thought and emotion. You have learned to free yourself from your (hidden) agenda.

4. You've taken time to **LOOK** at your position within the transaction of care, and ask yourself if you are the cause of something better or the effect of an other's situation or our broken system. You will learn to ask yourself am I reacting or am I responding? You know how to reframe your role in the patient encounter and your position in regards to your goal: to understand that the obstacles to your satisfaction aren't outside you, but within you. You know how to make the inner transformation and shift your position in your personal, internal quantum space from a negative to a positive one.

5. You've learned how to **EVALUATE** your situation by asking yourself, am I successful? Is my care making a difference for my patient? Am I feeling better as a result of caring for my patient? You can also recognize that you are feeling frustrated, your patient is frustrated, and neither of you are feeling satisfaction. In short, you know it is up to you to create your own experience—to create your world, moment by moment and you use the power you hold to do so.

6. Now you're ready to **CIRCLE BACK to the beginning**—to do it all again in every patient encounter and every colleague interaction. The lesson of step six is that you are never stuck! Whenever you're not feeling satisfied, you can go back to the beginning and see where you're disconnected from your original desire to care. And when

you *are* feeling satisfied, you can create fresh satisfaction for yourself and those around you by finding another to care for.

A Lesson from Junkyard Jake

As I found myself busier than ever, running faster and harder than ever, working more shifts in more challenging environments to support the process of writing and publishing the book, I was struggling emotionally with all that was going on. I was losing my certainty. I was not so certain that what I was writing in this book was going to be a game changer after all.

Then something very powerful happened. My dog Jake—"Junkyard Jake"—gave me an opportunity to experience another very powerful lesson about care.

Jake was an incredibly loving and sensitive dog. He was the runt of the litter and was challenged in so many ways since birth. In fact, the breeder was planning to put him down because she felt he would not be healthy. I could not allow that to happen, so twelve years ago, I adopted two dogs, Jake and his brother Max.

Jake was on borrowed time his whole life. He was very fragile and needed to be bottle-fed as a puppy. But throughout his life, he always looked after his brother. He cleaned Max's ears. He licked Max's wounds when he had his medial collateral ligament repaired. He let the kids tug on his ears and brush him. He let the smallest of them ride him like a pony. Every time he went outside he found a piece of junk to bring home to me as a present. He let me dress him up on holidays so we could have a new card to send to friends and family. He wore hats and sunglasses, bunny ears at Easter and reindeer antlers on Christmas.

In the dozen years I had the privilege to call Jake my own, he comforted me through each and every one of my disastrous personal dramas. The breeder was right, Jake did face a lot of health challenges, but he was always happy and he never complained. He did not cry about the eye problems that eventually took his sight. He did not whine about his mitral valve and the trouble he had breathing that resulted from congestive heart failure. He did not whimper about the water pills he had to swallow and all the trips he had to take outside because of them. He was always happy to see me, hang out with me and give me puppy kisses.

Jake was eighty-four years old—in dog years—when he developed a brain tumor. Although we did everything we could to extend his life, I knew his time was near. He was overcome by his health challenges and his happiness gave way to restlessness and discomfort. Max finally looked at me with eyes that said, "Do something to help him, please." On the way to the emergency veterinarian, Jake lost his cognition and began to seize. For the very first time in his life, it was very clear to me that he was suffering.

When we walked into the emergency clinic, they asked what was wrong. I was crying when I simply said my dog Jake needed to be euthanized. The response of the entire staff was so profoundly compassionate that even through my pain I could not help but notice. In a split second, everything softened and the hard edges blurred. I sensed these people knew exactly what Jake and I were going through. They spoke to me as if they knew us both, as if they had been there when we took those pictures for the holiday cards. They treated us with kindness, compassion, respect and reverence. It was as if something sacred from Heaven had descended and overtaken this piece of earth.

Their care made a difference for me, for Jake and for Jake's other daddy, Vince. The receptionist, the assistants and the vet herself all modeled back to me everything I had been writing in the book. It was as if they had *read* the book and were applying the framework, using the perspectives, insights and tools. They had all of my friends with them, Kindness, Compassion, Empathy, Sympathy, Caring, Sharing, Giving, along with Tolerance and, above all, Human Dignity. They cried with us, and they used those tears to make it better for all of us.

That experience could have been one of the most awful experiences of my life, but it was the best. It was the best because

I saw a new, a better, practice of medicine where care is just as important as cure. Where these heroes used the best stuff in their house of medicine and they included all of the best stuff that makes their house a home, all the energies of care, empathy and compassion. The stuff that gives Mom's chicken soup the power to heal; the stuff that makes Grandma's pickles taste best.

They used the energies of thought and emotion—exactly what's missing from the modern clinical professional delivery of goods and services we all call medicine. By adding these energetic quantum thought constructs to the physical goods and services we already provide, we can bring satisfaction back to the bedside, always. We can finally create satisfaction on both sides of the stethoscope.

What did I learn from Jake? That simply having the knowledge, perspective and tools is not enough. We have to commit to doing the work, every day. We have to engage in the process of continually regrouping: picking ourselves up, gathering our resources and circling back to the beginning where we'll apply step one all over again. We must see everything as an opportunity and dig in, to engage in the process of continuously creating satisfaction for ourselves, changing our world, making it better, one situation and one human encounter at a time.

Continuous Caring

The last chapter was all about recognizing what is going on inside our minds; it was filled with perspectives, insights and thoughts that you can inject into your mind to help you transform yourself internally. This internal transformation is what gives you the power to care whenever you need it. With the power to care, you can make a difference and change the reality you share with your patient. With the power to care, you can create satisfaction for both you and your patient. With the power to care you can heal your own compassion fatigue, empathetic overload and professional burnout.

Your power to care exists within your own mind. The trick—as you're discovering in this chapter—is that you don't just exercise the power to care once and change your reality for good. You need to go back to the beginning and apply the process afresh, whether you're already feeling satisfaction or whether you aren't.

When we recognize that we are not feeling satisfaction and consciously become aware of our own state of frustration, we are aware that we do not feel so good. This awareness that we are not feeling good exists in our mind, not our brain, but our "feeling bad" is "real," and it's part and parcel of what is going on in our brain as a result of the mix of neurotransmitters in our prefrontal cortex.

Awareness is in our mind and feeling bad is in our brain/body. Whenever we find ourselves feeling frustrated, we have the opportunity to move on to step six of our framework and circle back to the beginning and apply our framework to the situation we find ourselves in. Yes, we can do it all again: **remember** and reconnect to our desire to care, realize we must **earn** our own satisfaction, **formulate** our plan using the Perfect Equation and the six-step process for generating and delivering True Care, **look** at our position inside the transaction of care—are we the cause of something better?—and **evaluate** where our efforts have gotten us.

Even if we're not feeling frustrated—when we recognize we are satisfied, feeling good—the next step is still to circle back to the beginning, this time looking for another opportunity to care and create *more* satisfaction. Remember, satisfaction won't last in the moment unless we are actively creating more of it. This is how I make the best cup of coffee every time. Recognizing what we are feeling in real time requires us to consistently become conscious of the stream of thoughts running through our awareness. Our thoughts are constantly changing. We can control and transform what we are thinking and feeling by using our mind.

Why do we have to go back to step one even when we are feeling satisfied? Because the neurochemistry we have just created in our prefrontal cortex is dependent on neurotransmitters, which decay over time. A new thought will create a new neurochemistry that will cause us to feel good or bad, depending on the thought itself. If you think about this, you will see that you are now engaged in the process of practicing mind over matter. You are using your thoughts (energy) to control your brain's neurochemistry (matter).

What you have learned in this book is how to be the cause in any human encounter. When you are not aware of the stream of thoughts running through your system and you allow yourself to run on autopilot, your automatic reactions to your environment run the show. When you react automatically, you are the effect, not the cause. **When you choose to run on autopilot, you are always the effect of someone or something in your environment, something "out there."**

When you practice this framework we have been learning, you are engaging in the practice of causation. If you want to feel good more often, if you want to practice causation, using your mind to control matter, you will see that no matter what state you are experiencing—frustration or satisfaction, happiness or sadness, joy or depression—in order to be the cause of your satisfaction at any point in your day, you have no choice but move on and continue to transform and create your reality. You don't stop. You want to keep the energy flowing through you because whenever energy is flowing through you, you will feel good.

More satisfaction is not in the individual encounter. More satisfaction is in the continual process of giving care. You are now looking to be the cause of continuity. You are looking to be involved in a circular process where you are the cause of more and more feel-good moments at work. This is the circuitry of continuous satisfaction in the quantum world.

Your, my, biggest obstacle to success in the quantum world of care is going to be letting go of what we think we know, becoming aware of our stream of consciousness, turning off our autopilot and seeing what we have not been trained to see before. This is the only way we will be able to transcend our present limitations. Things in the quantum world often do not make sense, yet they have immense power. In medicine, most of us are logic-driven creatures, and as such we look to the end result and forget the process. Care in the quantum world is all about the process; it all depends on using the framework, remembering why we are here and what we want and connecting to our primary uncorrupted desire to care.

I have already shared experiences with you in the process of writing this book where I was not successful at choosing to apply the framework to create satisfaction in the emergency department in real time. Experiences where I had to search for days to find the way, the tool, the method to create satisfaction for myself when I was feeling nothing but frustrated. The goal of the framework is to help get us to the place where when we are feeling frustrated, we can flip a switch, and turn on the satisfaction, in real time, right now, every time: a continuous process of satisfaction continuously renewed.

A Better Day the Next Day

We have all heard of the concept of parallel universes. In each and every day, there are two days. We always have two choices. We can live the bad day, which ultimately leads to chaos, pain, suffering, decay, decline and depletion—or we can live the good day, but this will require heroic effort on our part.

Recently, I walked into work and we were double digits behind in triage with twenty-six patients in the lobby waiting to come back in to treatment rooms. We were getting hit hard with squad traffic as well. It was as busy and chaotic as it ever gets in any emergency department. Everyone was frustrated, and it felt as if I was in a room filled with a hundred angry complainers. No one was satisfied, no one was happy. Soon I was feeling the same. It was a very tough shift, but somehow we all made it through the night, all the patients got seen, and we turned over the department to day shift with a clean board. I left drained and exhausted, frustrated that I was not able to find satisfaction in what we were doing.

When I woke up from my nap the next day, I realized that I had a million chores to do before I could leave for work. I worked hard to complete them all and went back in to work without dinner, ready to face it again, hoping and praying that it would not be so busy and that I could escape my bad feelings and sense of overwhelm. But not long into the shift, something happened and my button, my "hey, what about me" button, got pushed by a police officer at the bedside of a violent patient. That was all it took. My sinister alter ego, Cranky Frankie, showed up and began to run the show.

I started complaining about everyone and everything. All I could see was the bad. Nothing was good. Even though I love the staff I work with, I could find nothing to appreciate in them. They were doing stupid things, not bringing the patients back to rooms fast enough, not taking orders off efficiently enough. There was no teamwork. There was no esprit de corps. I felt entitled to better.

Now, I know that entitlement is a death sentence. I know that the way to overcome entitlement is to appreciate. I tried to use the **TIME OUT** tool to stop, to inject new positive thoughts and emotions into my system and my environment, but I just could not connect with anything positive. Instead, I was allowing myself to be reactive and connecting with everything bad, wrong and negative in my environment. I knew that my negativity was only attracting more negativity. I knew that I was creating my own living, breathing hell. I knew that since my beast within, my Cranky Frankie, was automatically reacting to everyone and everything, I was actually injecting more negativity into my environment by speaking about it through complaining; complaining activates the negative forces in our environment. I know this.

I know inherently that the problem has nothing to do with the policemen, the nurse, the patient, the housekeeper or the secretary, but I was choosing to see them all as villains. Even though I know these people and know that they are all basically decent and competent, I was making the choice to extract only the bad from the situation. With my choice, I was cutting myself off from anything good. I *knew* this!

Our thoughts, both positive and negative, are manifested in our physical world through our words and then through our actions. Each and every one of us has some weakness or flaw, some button that, when pushed, causes us to see a situation as bad, then act out in some negative way. One of my go-to forms of negativity is to bad-mouth the situation and everyone in it.

There is a principle in quantum physics that can bring this all home. It states that through the act of watching, the observer affects what is being observed. Although Einstein was not able to prove this in his lifetime, researchers at the Weizmann Institute of Science have credibly documented the principle's validity. Their experiment, published in the journal *Nature*, clearly showed that what the observer believes will happen actually influences what does happen.

In the field of social sciences, we have learned the same thing. The "observer's paradox," so named by William Labov, essentially demonstrates that we will see what we expect to see. When we expect to see the bad, we connect to the bad and we live the bad day that ultimately leads us to being frustrated, problem-ridden, drained and exhausted. But when we do the hard and heroic work of injecting positivity, appreciation and enthusiasm into speaking, acting and seeing things differently, then we live the good day. Whether we are aware of it or not, we are creating our reality every day, moment to moment, by the choices we make in what to see.

Each and every one of us needs to ask ourselves, what is it that we actually see—what do we pay attention to—when our button is being pushed? We can then use this information to turn around the situation inside us, in our quantum inner space of our thoughts and emotions, so that we can escape the moment of living hell we are creating for ourselves and for those around us. But here is the catch; we will not automatically ask ourselves these questions. It doesn't happen instinctively; we have to make it happen.

That day, I was not successful. However, I was able to see what was going on in real time, then use this situation to regroup, go back through the framework and set myself up to have a better day the next day. We will all have days and moments when we don't succeed, but they will only be days and moments.

This happened to me, but it was just an event that happened one day. This is not the reality I live most days at work. I went back to the framework and did the quantum work to transform it. All the work I have done and the work I continue to do gives me the energy that I need to take myself back, over and over again, to the land of quantum satisfaction. These events and days will happen to you too. They happen to everyone who chooses to swallow the blue pill of self-responsibility. This does not mean that our framework does not always work—it does. Using the **TIME OUT** tool to stop and allow yourself to transform internally is a conscious choice, and it will always be difficult. But the best news is that the more difficult it is and the harder we have to work to see it differently, the greater the satisfaction, happiness and joy we will be able to create for ourselves.

Chapter 10

Restore and Renew

Well, here we are. We've made it to the end of our hero's journey. I have shared everything I have learned and everything I know about care, how to connect to it, how to create it, how to give it and how to effectively deliver it. That's all I've got. You now have all the tools, insight, perspective and tactical information you need to step onto the floor in the hospital and create satisfaction on both sides of the stethoscope.

The hallmark of the hero's journey, though, is that the hero travels into the unknown—delves deep into the dark places without and within—and returns to the ordinary world transformed. My ultimate goal is for both you and me to be transformed in the same way—to become so accomplished at this process of creating what we want that we feel satisfied most, if not all, of the time, both at work and in our personal lives. In other words, my prayer is that by using our seven-step framework in our own personal lives and situations, we can transcend our present limitations and live happier, more fulfilled lives both inside and outside the hospital.

Let's look one more time at all the steps on this path of ours:

1. Now you **REMEMBER** what you came here for in the first place, and you've reconnected to your desire to care, to make a difference, to make patients feel better *because* you care.

2. You've realized that you are responsible for creating your own satisfaction, and if you are going to feel good, you have to shift your focus from the physical components of cure to the intangible energies of care. You know that only you can **EARN** your satisfaction for yourself.

3. You have learned to **FORMULATE** your plan for getting the satisfaction you crave that comes from caring. You have recalculated the transaction of care according to the Perfect Equation, by which your giving True Care and your patient's receiving your True Care add up to the energy of satisfaction in the quantum world of thought and emotion. You have learned to free yourself from your (hidden) agenda.

4. You've taken time to **LOOK** at your position within the transaction of care, and ask yourself if you are the cause of something better or the effect of another's situation. You know to ask yourself, am I reacting or am I responding? You know how to reframe your role in the patient encounter and your position in regards to your goal: to understand that the obstacles to your satisfaction aren't outside you, but within you. You know how to make the inner transformation and shift your position in your personal, internal quantum space from a negative to a positive one.

5. You've learned to **EVALUATE** your situation by asking yourself, am I successful? Is my care making a difference for my patient? Am I feeling better as a result of caring for my patient? You can also recognize that you are feeling frustrated, your patient is frustrated, and neither of you are feeling satisfaction. In short, you know it is up to you to create your own experience—to create your world, moment by moment and you use the power you hold to do so.

6. You can always **CIRCLE BACK to the beginning**—start all over again in every patient encounter and every colleague interaction. You now know that you are never stuck! Whenever you're not feeling satisfied, you can go back to the beginning and see where you're disconnected from your

original desire to care. And when you *are* feeling satisfied, you can create fresh satisfaction for yourself and those around you by finding another to care for.

7. Now you're ready to take the last step on this hero's journey—here you will learn new ways to **TAKE CARE** of yourself, to restore and renew yourself by applying the quantum skills you've learned to energize and elevate every part of your life. This is where we invest energy in maintaining our "equipment"—our physical and energetic caring systems. We continue to change internally, which gives us the power to transcend our present limitations and change not only ourselves but the world around us as well. We become fully realized, fully satisfied caregivers—and, better yet, fully realized, satisfied and happy human beings.

Who We Want to Be

To achieve lasting satisfaction, we must ask ourselves, why don't we have enough of what we want? For me, at work, in the hospital, behind the stethoscope, my desire was to care for patients, and I wanted that care to make things better. I was working so hard for these people; why were they not satisfied? And why did I feel so flat, empty and frustrated?

That night when I lay on the dirty floor of the emergency department, being choked by my larger-than-life patient in the midst of his psychotic rage, was only the beginning for me of an intensely personal process of introspection and self-discovery. I did not realize anything that night while I was being strangled, but my internal processing of the "happening," and the other frustrations and failures I had experienced as both a patient and a doctor, added a new dimension to my life journey. I was fully focused on my unfolding experiences and insights around caring for and being cared for, and this contemplation continued over the next two years as I worked to solve these riddles—for myself as well as for you.

I have shared my journey of self-discovery with you throughout this book. It began with my wanting more from life. Although that dirty emergency room floor was a punctuation point, the journey continued through all of the research I did to define care and figure out what it would take to deliver care so that I would be able to actualize my desire to make a difference and change the world.

The journey continued through the writing of this book, which was a labor of love designed to actualize my desire to care for *you*. I just had to help those I work with—the entire community of medical, nursing and paramedical professionals across the globe, all those who suffer from the occupational hazard of compassion fatigue and burnout—to help you understand what care really is, and I had to give you the tools you need to be able to care effectively and find the satisfaction you crave. It turns out that caring effectively has an even more important fringe benefit. In our connecting to and stepping into another's pain, then turning on our own compassion for others we find our only protection from compassion fatigue, professional burn out and the resultant loss of our own humanity.

But the journey does not stop there, because satisfaction is not only intangible, it is fleeting and ever-expanding. What satisfies us today will not satisfy us tomorrow, because we will want more. We will still want more from our lives and our careers, even if we all become masters at using the framework I've laid out in this book for creating and experiencing satisfaction on both sides of the stethoscope.

You see, once we are satisfied, we will still want more, and we will not want more of the same thing. We will want more new, more fresh, more novel and ever better experiences of satisfaction. As humans we are hard-wired to care, and we are hard-wired to continuously want something better. Physiologically and energetically, humans can never feel fulfilled or fully actualized when we settle for anything. When we settle, we always get less than what we thought we were settling for.

There is a disparity between what we have and what we want. There is a disparity between who we are and *who we want to be*. This is a disparity between who we are now and who we would be if we were to actualize our full potential. Almost all of the sadness, depression or emptiness we feel in our lives exists because of this disparity—because of the fact that we are not yet who we aspire to be.

This is not exactly new information. Humans have known about this for quite a long time. There is a Native American legend about a grandfather speaking to his grandson, who is angry because a friend hurt him. He tells his grandson that he has been angry too.

This wise elder goes on to tell the boy that there is a "fight" going on inside of him, a terrible fight between two wolves. One wolf is anger, envy, sorrow, regret, greed, arrogance, self-pity, guilt, resentment, inferiority, lies, false pride, superiority and ego. The other wolf is joy, peace, love, hope, serenity, humility, kindness, benevolence, empathy, generosity, truth, compassion and faith. He tells his grandson that the same fight is going on inside the boy and each and every other person too. His grandson asks him, "Which wolf wins, Grandfather?" He replies, "The wolf you choose to feed."

None of us wants to feed the wrong wolf. We all want to be great doctors, great nurses, great mothers, great fathers, great brothers and sisters. We all want to be great people. We all want to be the best possible version of ourselves in any given moment. Earlier in the book I told you that people do not get out of bed in the morning, look in the mirror and say, *I am going to hold back today, do less than I am capable of.*

Man as a species is evolving. The times they are a-changing. To many, it is becoming obvious that the purpose of our lives is to bring these two selves, the present limited self and the best possible self that we aspire to be, closer together in any given moment and over time. This is the process of becoming self-actualized, happy, powerful and satisfied with who we are.

Free Will and Your Brain

In healthcare, and in all the service professions, we came to our jobs because we have a desire to care. When we care effectively, we generate satisfaction for both ourselves and others. True caring requires us to delay our own gratification in the moment, put our own needs aside for a moment, and put the needs of another in front of our own. When we care effectively for others and change things for them, we feel satisfied.

Satisfaction is much different from pleasure. Pleasure is a physical sensation. Satisfaction is both a physical and an energetic phenomenon. It is an enduring happiness or fulfillment that contains a sense of accomplishment. Pleasure and instant gratification are almost synonymous, but satisfaction actually requires us to delay our pleasure—to use our free will to delay our gratification. You can do this! Let's face it, none of us would have made it through medical school, nursing school or any school, for that matter, if we were not able to delay gratification with our free will.

We learned in medical and nursing school that at each and every moment of our lives, all sorts of automatic neurochemical reactions are happening unconsciously and involuntarily in all the cells and synapses in our brain. Different functions are located in different anatomical areas of our brain. The prefrontal cortex is the most thoughtful, feeling part of our brain. It controls the functions of forethought, judgment, impulse control, organization, planning, learning from past choices and missteps. Empathy, compassion and insight are also found here. Many refer to this lobe of our neuroanatomy as "The Executive," because it acts like the boss. It is the place where decisions and choices are made.

Humans have the largest amount of prefrontal cortex of all the species on our planet, and the prefrontal cortex is where our free will, our power to choose, resides. We humans are the only animal with the unique power of free will. We can't help having our automatic physiologic reactions to stimuli in our environment—it's eons of evolution we are fighting against—but with our free will, our power to choose, we have the ability to interrupt the animal-like reactions of our beast within.

Dr. Daniel Amen, a neurologist who is considered an expert in the clinical interpretation of brain imaging in modern science, tells us that the prefrontal cortex is also where our conscience resides. I find it fascinating that, looked at a certain way, the word *con-science* literally means to go against physiology. Dr. Amen believes that this is the place where our brain's cellular physiology and neurochemistry intersect with the thoughts in our mind. In other words, this is the crux of our mind-body connection. Here, the thoughts in our mind affect the cells in the grey matter in our brain, which is where we get the popular saying "mind over matter" that you've heard throughout this book.

Each and every day, our physical five-sense system brings our brain way too much information for our brains to process. Nothing is more important to any organism than its own survival, so it makes sense that this information comes directly and indirectly into one of the most ancient and primordial parts of the brain: the amygdala, about the size of an almond, straddling the brainstem as the innermost part of the temporal lobes. The primary function of the amygdala is to sort through all of that information coming into the brain, looking for anything in our immediate environment that might harm us. It is a danger detector.

The amygdala is part of the limbic system, which performs many activities, most having to do with control of functions necessary for self-preservation and preservation of the species. It is part of the autonomic nervous system and the endocrine system and is intimately connected to reactions to emotional stimuli and memory. Your amygdala gives you the ability to feel emotions and perceive emotions in other people. It plays a big part in arousal, motivation and reinforcing behaviors. Some refer to the limbic system as the reactive and feeling brain, in contrast to the cerebral cortex, which is often referred to as the thinking brain.

Our amygdala is in constant and close communication with our five senses and our internal organs, including our adrenal glands; it's responsible for the dry mouth, rapid heart rate and tense muscles in our freeze-fight-or-flee responses to danger. In today's modern society, this internal system of ours is also now responsible for our feeling stress, with all the detrimental effects of excessive cortisol production that go along with it. This system is also physically responsible for our physiologic autopilot emotional reactions in our interpersonal encounters with others, including our clinical patient encounters.

Our limbic system does not always operate in our best interests when our challenges and choices are more complex than running away from a saber-toothed tiger. In our stressful society, and even more so in our stressful positions within the emergency department or hospital, when the volume and the acuity of patients are high, when there are so many things on our to-do list and we are running out of time, we can start to physically feel stress because of the biochemicals that prime our bodies to fight, flee or freeze.

When we are so hyperstimulated by our environment, we often start to feel like we are losing control. This is when our limbic system is automatically activated and we can find it oh so difficult to "keep it together." This process is automatic, physiologic, biological and mammalian. Modern-day stressors activate the system, and cortisol, adrenalin and other chatecholamines are generated. When the amount of stress reaches a critical point, even the smallest challenge can trigger an automatic reaction, an amygdala reaction, a knee-jerk reaction, where instead of caring for those around us, we act like a jerk.

This automatic, physiologic system, running just under our conscious awareness, is human and none of us are immune to it. Social scientists in the past decade have named this process emotional hijacking. What is so awful about it is that as we work to become the best versions of ourselves we are constantly being hijacked by our own physiology. As we struggle to feed the good wolf inside, our limbic system is automatically nourishing our bad wolf. A piece of our brain that is about the size and shape of an almond is working against us and our efforts to be better and do better. Seriously, Houston, we have a big (or an almond-sized) problem here! The high catecholamine states generated by our amygdala actually diminish function of the higher cortex, where the power of our free will and "con-science" resides.

We are not in a position to control our environment or the amount of stress it will induce in us, so the only control we have, if we are looking for happiness, satisfaction or fulfillment in our jobs and lives, is to control our own thoughts and behaviors. If we want to be successful at giving care, we need a tool that will allow us to shut down our automatic physiologic reactive system at will. Well, we already have the tool! The **TIME OUT** tool I have shared with you allows us to, in effect, shut down that aspect of our physiology. This is the only way we can exercise our innate and uniquely human power of free will to give care regardless of what is going on externally in our environment. In medicine we are always controlling or changing physiology—the patho-physiology of disease. Just knowing that it's not yourself but your physiology that you're fighting to control gives you the power to change it.

I am reminding you here of the limbic system and that little sliver of the temporal lobe called the amygdala and the way all of this affects our physiology so that we can use that knowledge as we move through our lives with more peace and more energy and create ever more feel-good moments. Remember, the goal is to escape the effects of our stressors, to transform internally, and then create our own feel-good moments and satisfying experiences. Practicing our seven-step framework is not, let me repeat, IS NOT a natural or automatic thing; it takes real effort. Having a knee-jerk reaction and engaging in any of the negative behaviors that go along with it—complaining, avoiding others, judging others, feeling entitled, gossiping, manipulating—THAT is automatic.

Falling into one of those reactions requires no conscious effort and does not really engage our power to choose, to exercise our free will. The reason heroic effort is required to put our framework into practice is that it pushes us against and beyond our nature, our physiology. Executing the framework successfully requires us to use our free will by using the thoughts in our mind, using our conscious awareness to change the chemistry in our frontal and prefrontal cortex.

Bear in mind, we want the feeling that comes from knowing that our efforts to care actually make things better. The feeling we want is contained within the intangible energies of thoughts and emotion. These exist in Einstein's unseen quantum world where everything is relative and nothing is linear. While we may not be able to detect these energies with our physical senses, we swim in a world of energies all the time. As long as we are breathing, thinking and feeling, we are creating energies that are broadcast into our environment.

Let's look at another way our automatic physiology works to sabotage our efforts to get what we want.

The Mood Mirror

Ever notice how we feel happy around happy people, sad around depressed people or even agitated when we are around anxious people? Why and how does this happen automatically? There is a human process, active from infancy, that causes us to imitate the facial expressions, postures and voices of the people around us. Different expressions trigger certain moods, the same moods experienced by the person we mimic. The process happens so fast that we have no conscious awareness of it. An interconnected network of cells in the brain that make up the Mirror Neuron System, or MNS, governs this mimicry of ours.

According to David R. Hamilton, PhD, the MNS is a bit like a high-definition camera that observes and records every detail of people's facial expressions, body language, pupil movements and even vocal tones. It works wherever you go: Paul Ekman, a PhD at the University of California–San Francisco, has discovered that the facial expressions for seven emotions—anger, fear, sadness, disgust, surprise, contempt and happiness—are the same across all cultures around the world. So if you are hanging out with someone who is happy, and their happiness is written all over their face, so to speak, your MNS will record their displays of happiness, but it will also signal the same displays in you. Your MNS gives you the power to know what others are feeling! In other words, your MNS will then activate the muscles in your face and generate a smile, which will then create endorphins that make you feel happier too.

However, in the quantum world of energy, negativity exists as well, so we are just as likely to catch someone's bad mood and negative attitude. And given the fact that our patients in the emergency department are often anxious, frightened, depressed, sad or even angry, we are swimming in some big negativity. Worse yet, as we all know intuitively even without the brain science, a negative co-worker can pollute the entire department and create an even more toxic work environment. A negative physician or charge nurse can make work miserable for all of us.

So what can we do? How can we stop ourselves from being infected? There is no way for us to turn off or disable our MNS. It runs in the background, just under our awareness, all the time, in every human interaction during our day.

First of all, knowledge is power. Simply being aware that we have a Mirror Neuron System functioning 24/7 can help us understand how negativity in our environment affects our mood. When we see a co-worker acting out, we can offer a more positive solution. If he continues to act out, we can ask him to stop before we allow him to infect us. If he can't stop, we can choose to walk away. We can make it a personal rule not to participate in the negative behaviors of others.

More importantly, we can reconnect with our original, pure, uncorrupted desire to care and to make a difference for others. Our desire to care will allow us to embrace the MNS, for it allows us to be empathetic and feel what our patients, their families and our co-workers are feeling. When we connect to them and feel their pain, their distress, their disease, we can choose to feel compassion for them. Then all the positive feel-good dopamine centers in our prefrontal cortex will light up, and we will be able to speak or act from there and say or do something positive that will change things for them. We can broadcast our care, our compassion and our pure desire to make things better into our energetic environment by staying positive, happy and enthusiastic about our mission.

When we find a way to stay positive, we can slowly but surely improve the mood and morale of the entire department. Our co-workers will become more resilient and more able to generate the caring thoughts and emotions *they* need to be effective givers of care. What we think matters. How we feel matters. All the positive energy we share or give away to others in our environment really makes a difference.

By now, we know that we feel happy when our prefrontal cortex drips with dopamine. I have said it over and over again. Humans are hard-wired to care. Our prefrontal cortex drips with dopamine when we feel compassion for another. Turns out this feel-good dopamine actually activates the learning centers of the brain, allowing our brain to take advantage of its inherent neuroplasticity and remodel itself, creating new neural pathways that allow us to develop more of our full potential in terms of intelligence, athletic ability, musicality, creativity and productivity. (More on neuroplasticity a little later.)

What are some other ways to get the dopamine flowing? Research has shown that you can prime people to become more altruistic by giving them something small yourself. Priming a four-year-old by asking her to remember her most happy time actually causes her spatial memory to increase dramatically, allowing her to put blocks together up to 50 percent faster than children who were not primed. Doctors primed to be positive come to the correct diagnosis 19 percent faster than doctors primed to be negative. When primed to be optimistic, salespeople have 37 percent higher levels of sales. Turns out happiness itself confers a significant performance advantage on all humans.

In this regard I highly recommend Shawn Achor's best-selling book *The Happiness Advantage*. Shawn, who is at Harvard and considered an expert in his field, has some great ideas for boosting your level of happiness in the moment and over time. Research has shown that writing five things down on paper that you can be grateful for each morning increases your baseline happiness for twenty-four hours. If you do this for twenty-one days, the effects continue for six months. This is because your brain is devoting more resources to looking for good things as opposed to stressors and hassles. You are functioning higher in the cortex and less near the brainstem. You actually get better at navigating your life with this simple thirty-second intervention.

He also tells us that journaling for three minutes about a positive experience each day for thirty days caused participants in the study to experience 50 percent fewer trips to the doctor's office. These people also showed improvements in their immune system function and reported being more social. Research has demonstrated that exercise is as effective as antidepressants in improving positive mood and that meditation really does work to cause physical changes in the body. A simple meditation such as following your breath changes the measured electrical activity in the brain and increases the number of gamma waves. Those who meditate this way have better insight, and this is what allows them to experience the "aha" moment more readily.

Success is more likely if you use your ability to positively adapt to the world. Being happy or positive allows us to be more optimistic and see stress as a challenge rather than a threat. One of the best investments we can make is in a supportive social network of friends and colleagues. Life is like a lab where we experiment with different sorts of creative processes until we find the one that works for us, the process that fulfills our desires and results in happiness.

My entire journey started with being unhappy with what I had. I said I want more! I said that I want more from this life! There has to be more to life than this! Now that we have our seven-step framework, we are no longer slaves to our physiology. We now have a new choice. We can delay our gratification in the instant and do the work of creating lasting fulfillment and quantum levels of satisfaction by creating win-win solutions that change everything for everybody.

When we are feeling less than satisfied, feeling bad or frustrated, and the stress is spiraling upward, we can pause and then open ourselves to lifting ourselves up and out of the stress by injecting something positive. It was Dr. Shaun Marler who said, "To get something you've never had, you have to do something you have never done." Now we know that we can stop, use the **TIME OUT** tool, and, with our free will to choose our thoughts, take the opportunity to inject some new and positive thoughts from our mind into our prefrontal cortex. We can change the physiology of our brain and create something different.

By controlling our thoughts, we now control ourselves, and we can actually have some real control over our physiology, the situation and the environment. We are no longer victims of anything or anybody. This is the practice of being the cause. This is the technology of mind over matter.

This is not natural. This is not automatic. This requires huge amounts of conscious effort. But practicing this framework is what will allow us to be great doctors, great nurses, great medics, great lovers, great partners, great fathers, great mothers, great brothers and great sisters, and this is what will allow us to become the great people we so want to be. This is the way we get what we really want. This is our transformation from ordinary to extraordinary.

The High Life

Practicing our seven-step framework is how we eliminate the disparity between what we have (frustration and burnout) and what we want (feeling good and real and lasting satisfaction). When we begin to practice, we are better prepared to be successful if we remember that this process is not natural or automatic. This is a process we use to go against our mammalian nature, our animal-like physiologic/biologic ancient internal physical processes.

In the hospital, when we are working so hard and we feel no appreciation and get no thank you, we often want instant relief, but the truth of the matter is, instant relief only delays the realization of our goals. We will have to do the things that we do not like to do, those things that do not come easy. Often, even with all of our education and training and our feeling that we deserve respect, we will have to humble ourselves and be sensitive to others who have less understanding than we do. We will need to be kind to those who are disrespecting us. We will have to find creative ways to be caring to those who are less fortunate. We will have to go against our physiology. Our nature is to care; our physiology gets in the way. This working against our own automatic physiology is the only way to generate the payoff we are looking for.

I know this sounds so hard that it borders on the impossible, but I have really great news. There is a whole new exciting field of study in neuroscience today that focuses on neuroplasticity. These scientists and clinicians are discovering the ways in which we can rewire our brains. We used to think that things like personality and intelligence were fixed by a certain age. We now know this not the case. We can change ourselves. We can control our brain with our mind. We can practice mind over matter right now, even if we don't have all the scientific details worked out.

So far what we do know about neuroplasticity is that we can rewire our brains by using conscious focus and attention along with new experiences (training). We can effectively use our thoughts (our mind, not our brain) to overcome our past conditioning. Hence the new battle cry: Change your thoughts, change your brain, change (y)our world! This may become the new definition of "will power."

There is a war going on inside of us, between the two wolves, or between our pleasure centers (our inner child) and our prefrontal cortex (our adult, thoughtful part of our brain). Our pleasure centers are driven by our spoiled inner child, who wants what it wants, NOW. No matter the consequence. Our inner child is looking to feed our pleasure centers with the toy, the puppy, the cake, the alcohol, the heroin, the Vicodin, the Valium, the cigarette, the gambling, the shaming of another, the manipulation of another, the punching another in the nose or whatever it is in the moment that will stimulate or feed those pleasure centers and bring instant relief from the stress imposed on the system by our environment through the limbic system and the amygdala. Left untamed, this little beast within will run amok and ruin our lives.

In order to exercise our free will, we have to become aware of what is already going on inside us automatically, stop it and shut it down. We can then inject a new thought that will allow us to ditch our automatic reaction and respond instead by making the conscious choice to do or say something different. In order to be successful people and successful caregivers, it is imperative that we strengthen our prefrontal cortex, that we reshape the neural pathways we find there. It is imperative, if we are going to be really successful adults, that we are able to put our inner child into time out. We know we can do this because of all of the exciting emerging scientific findings coming from the field of neuroplasticity. The **TIME OUT** tool is the first step in the reshaping of our neural pathways.

Using the **TIME OUT** tool to interrupt your automatic physiologic mammalian system will allow you to have something new come out of you. This will allow me to have something new come out of me. Instead of punching the arch-villain in the nose, we will be able to create a win-win solution. Let me explain what I mean and how this ties into our own personal evolution as humans as well as the overall elevation of all of humanity.

The very first step in our framework is reconnecting to our desire. In other words, what do we want or feel we need in the moment? Science, psychology and medicine have been trying to answer this question forever. Over time the answers have changed, but out of all of the attempts to answer this question, Abraham Maslow's work done in the 1950s remains valid today for understanding human motivation and personal development.

His work is usually represented by a pyramid and understood as a hierarchy of needs, with the most basic needs at the bottom of the pyramid and the higher needs closer to the top. Originally, the needs from bottom to top were physiological, safety, love or belonging, esteem and self-actualization. Starting at the base of the pyramid, we go from food, water, air, sleep and sex to bodily security, employment, resources, morality, family, health and prosperity. Moving upward, we find intimate friends, sexual intimacy and strong family connections, then self-esteem, confidence, achievement, and respect of others and from others. Finally, at the top, we find creativity, spontaneity, problem solving, transcendence and realizing our full potential.

Since the Industrial Revolution, especially in Western civilizations, many of man's needs have been not only met but exceeded. We live in an abundant society, and once you get beyond man's physiologic, social and economic needs, our needs and desires become more and more personal. Today, most feel that humans living in such an abundant society have universal needs for certainty (meaning comfort or the ability to avoid pain and have pleasure), uncertainty (meaning variety or surprise), significance or meaning, connection or love, and growth and contribution beyond the self.

In our present society and our evolving world economy, these needs play out very differently than they used to. As a result, we now have three choices when it comes to the way in which we live our lives. We can live the low life, the comfortable life or the high life. Which life we live depends on which level of our neurochemistry or anatomy we operate from.

Stimulus-response animals have no choice. They are limited to reacting to the challenges placed in front of them by their environment. They are not really making conscious choices. They are just doing whatever it takes to get by. When humans live this way, they are living the low life. I call this the low life because they are functioning within the lower levels of their brain, neurochemistry and physiology.

This sort of functioning is a requirement when humans do not live in an abundant society where all their basic needs are met. If you need food, you must do whatever is necessary to get food. You are controlled by your animal-like drives for food, water, shelter, safety, affection and sex. When we live the low life, we really have no voice or influence in the world.

As Western society progressed into the modern age, humans looked to fill their higher needs with consumerism and were motivated primarily to have more and more of the good things in life. This led to living what I call the comfortable life.

In the comfortable life, we are looking for stuff and our motivation is extrinsic. I relearned this lesson when I recovered from cancer and worked so hard to have everything this life had to offer. I had the best house, the best job, the best car, the best dogs, the best partner, the best of the best, but I was never more empty. The problem with this comfortable life is that there is no happiness or fulfillment here beyond the stuff we accumulate.

When we are living the comfortable life, we are operating within the brainstem and the cortex and using some, but not all, of our prefrontal cortex. We make decisions based on our free will, but they arise from our extrinsic motivations for more respect, more money, more security, more success and more stuff to prove we are successful.

When we are living the comfortable life, we are using our mind and we do have consciousness, but we begin to feel that something just isn't right; we are not engaged with our stuff. We do have power and influence in our world, but we begin to ask ourselves, *Is this really what life is all about? What is it that I am all about? What is it that I stand for? What is really important in life? What do I want to use my power and influence for?* We start to wonder what is the legacy we will leave in this world.

Of all the human needs, only two, the need for personal growth and the need for contribution beyond the self, will bring lasting fulfillment or satisfaction. And this is where many of us find ourselves now with the collapse of the world economy, which was primarily consumer-driven and based on the accumulation of stuff, power and control. Eleanor Roosevelt was ahead of her time when she distinguished the high life this way: "Great minds discuss ideas; average minds discuss events; small minds discuss people." The times they are a-changing, and what satisfied us yesterday no longer holds any meaning or value for us now. Everyone everywhere is looking for ideas and searching for answers. This is leading many to live a new sort of life, what I call the high life.

The individual living the high life is functioning on all levels of his neuroanatomy and physiology. In addition, he chooses to take full advantage of his uniquely human free will. He recognizes that his conscious awareness of the thoughts in the mind (which are of a higher order than any function in the brain) is of paramount importance. His choosing which thoughts to engage gives him the ultimate control. He uses his conscious choice like a scalpel and cuts out any negative and destructive thoughts.

This individual is no longer competing against others, she's competing with herself, setting the bar ever higher. She is no longer worried about the car the Joneses are driving and she is not interested in getting one up on the Joneses by buying the next model up. She is no longer extrinsically motivated; her motivation comes from within. These people have real power and influence in the world and they are asking themselves, *Am I living my fully authentic life? Am I living the best possible version of myself in my life?*

The conscious human living the high life is setting his own challenges, truly responding to life. The conscious human living the high life is challenging himself to live a *better* life. These people are using novelty and challenge to retrain their brains, taking advantage of the science of neuroplasticity to consciously design the experience of their life. Their desire to contribute beyond the self, for creative expression of their innermost authentic self, their quest for more from life, opens them up and fills them with wisdom and meaning, no matter what is going on around them.

Those living the high life, the conscious life, are looking for ways to bring what already exists inside of them into the world so that they can see their own essence, their intrinsic goodness and higher qualities, reflected back to them through others and in the world. It is sort of like the process Michelangelo talked about when he was asked how he created the famous statue of David. He said he chipped away at the rock until the David that was already in the rock was revealed.

Tools for Transformation

So how do we move from the comfortable life, where happiness does not exist, to the high life, where there are inordinate amounts of lasting happiness, satisfaction, meaning, purpose and abundance? They say that the path to hell is paved with good intentions, and we must always remember this if we want to create heaven on earth. When we are looking for change in our lives, we cannot substitute thought or talk for action.

We all know we should exercise, but we don't. When it comes to exercise, then, we have fallen into the knowing-doing gap. Simply talking about it does nothing, changes nothing and definitely creates nothing. Brooding about how messed up things are, or how messed up we are, fat, unhealthy, stuck in a bad job or relationship—this is not action. Thinking or dreaming about change is not change. Action is the only way out of where we are now. Action is the only way out of *who* we are now.

We all know this intuitively. One day, a person who is unfit, out of shape and overweight wakes up and decides, *No more. I will be fit, healthy and sexy.* Once people reach this point, they then move through a creative process where they hate to exercise, they can't stand it, they go to the gym, they are humiliated by their appearance, they hate the exercise, they suffer through it, and then they start to see results—and as they become healthier and more fit, more lean, more sexy, more accomplished at exercise, one day they realize that they are now addicted to exercise. They don't feel good if they don't do it. They can't live without it.

How did this happen? They challenged themselves, they went to their consciousness and used their free will. They went against their nature (their physiology, their neurochemistry), they stepped out of their comfort zone, they did not accept or settle for instant gratification, they kept their eye on a more positive future. They pressed the pause button, left their old patterned conditioning and started operating on a higher level.

As a result, the gym, which used to be a source of failure and humiliation, began to nourish them, to feed them, to be a place where they revealed their inner beauty, where they chipped away at the rock until their inner David was revealed. This process brings them lasting satisfaction through challenge, accomplishment, hard work and effort. Now their physiology—their neurochemistry, their limbic system, their amygdala, their cortex and their prefrontal cortex, their beast within—is working for them rather than against them.

To accomplish this, you have to use the **TIME OUT** tool, run to your consciousness and stop your behavior, shut down your reactive automatic neurochemical and physiological system, and suspend time for yourself, just long enough to realize that your desire may not be manifest in this moment. Allow this to be the case. Ask yourself, *How can I manifest my desire? What action can I perform right now that will move me closer to the me I want to be, to the results I want to see?* This is how you can take control of your automatic mammalian physiology and transcend your present limitations.

At the risk of being redundant, our dissatisfaction comes from the fact that we are not living our highest life, that there is still a disparity between who we are now and who we want to be. We have the opportunity to ask ourselves, *Who is it that I want to be and what actions do I need to take to get me there?* Now I would like to make this practical and actionable.

We all have day timers, smart phones, computers or even note pads that contain lists upon lists of things to do. We actually call them "to-do" lists. Realize this once and for all: to-do lists do not grow you as a person, nor do they help you manifest your highest potential or your best self. Go ahead, take out your to-do list and pick any task on it. Ask yourself, *Does this action propel me towards the person I want to be?* We do not need any more to-do lists.

What we actually need are three lists. The first and most important list is the "To Be" or the "To Become" list. The type of thing to place on this list is anything that completes the sentence "I want to be_____." Happy, lean and sexy, caring, sharing, a loving wife, a great mother, a business tycoon, a body builder, whatever you want to be, put it on the list.

The second list is the "Required Transformative Actions" list. If you want to be a loving wife, then you need to take an action that will demonstrate your love for your husband—whatever that means for you. If you want to be a great mother, you need take an action that will show you to be a great mother.

The third list is what we used to call our to-do list, but it is now called the "Chores and Responsibilities" list. Going to the bank to deposit your check is a chore; it will not make you a business tycoon. Taking a class on business at your local community college or online is an action you could take to bring you closer to being a business tycoon.

Here's an example:

TO BECOME	REQUIRED TRANSFORMATIVE ACTION
Healthy	Learn about nutrition
	Eat a specific diet
	45 minutes of cardio 5 times a week
A loving mother	Schedule a trip to the zoo for your five-year-old surprise him by picking him up early from schoc
	Make Friday FAMILY NIGHT
	Serve special dinners and create activities for y family to enjoy
A great doctor or nurse	Buy and read *BACK FROM BURNOUT* -
	Apply the R.E.F.L.E.C.T framework to your life
Amazing	Do something amazing!
CHORES AND RESPONSIBILITIES	
Pick up the laundry	
Get the oil changed	
Pay the bills	
Buy the groceries	

Change is not instantaneous: as you use these three lists to manage your life, look forward to a new you, a new life, and realize that things change slowly until they change completely. Our To Become list now is the organizing principle of our day and the central experience of our life. Working on your To Become list automatically moves *you* up on your list of priorities.

First we decide who or what we want to be, then we take the actions that are required and do whatever is necessary to move us closer to who it is we want to be(come). Finally, we do our chores and take care of our responsibilities. These three lists work well to transition us from the comfortable life to the high life. They work in concert with each other, using tactical information to transform us so that we can transcend our previous limitations, making us grander people who are more capable of actualizing our desires. This is empowering. This feels good. This is creating lasting quantum levels of satisfaction.

As we progress, our To Become list and our Required Transformative Action list will change with us. Our chores and responsibilities will pretty much remain the same. Using these lists, and applying our seven-step framework to our own lives and any situation in our life, is what will restore us and renew us so that we can be the healthcare heroes we want to be. Using these lists will allow us "to be(come)" the people our patients, our co-workers, our families, our community, our society and the world need us to be. We will lead everyone to the world of quantum satisfaction through our actions of care. We will make a difference and we will change our world.

Everyone coming into the hospital expects to find care. But we are the only ones who can generate that care. So we must take care of ourselves, do everything we can to restore and renew. We can strive to generate and carry happiness around with us all day long. This happiness is our energetic immune system, and this will keep us safe from emotional contagion and hijacking! Aristotle said, "Happiness is the meaning and the purpose of life, the whole aim and end of human existence."

So ask yourself, do you feel good? What exactly are you doing to make yourself feel good? Remember, action is the only way out of where we are now. Action is the only way out of who we are now. As caregivers, we are particularly bad at self-care. Our selfless nature does not serve us well in the long run if we do not find a way to care for, and invest our benevolent energies into, ourselves.

Investing in ourselves, taking the time and putting the effort into self-restoration when we are outside the hospital, is an absolute must for the modern hero of healthcare. This kind of self-care is vitally important, for we need stamina and strength to do the physical work of cure and the quantum work of care.

I have found that my days are much more challenging if I haven't taken the time to rest and take care of myself. At the simplest of levels, it is hard to care for others if you are tired or hungry. So start with the basics. Pay attention to your sleep patterns. We all do shift work, so pick a time of the day where you can always be asleep. Anchor your sleep to that time.

Learn to respect the sleep cycle, which takes ninety minutes to complete for all humans, no exceptions. Sleep in increments of ninety minutes, so an hour and a half, three hours, four and a half hours, six hours or seven and a half hours. Trust me, I am a doctor, I have been doing shift work and working holidays and off hours my whole life. The research does not lie—sleep this way and you will feel much better.

Once you have the basics covered, invest in yourself. Exercise, take classes, read, engage in volunteer work you find meaningful or take time to mentor others with what you have learned here. Make an effort to move from the comfortable life, where lasting satisfaction and happiness is impossible, to living the high life, where you are the creator of your own life, your own satisfaction, your own purpose and meaning and personal sense of happiness and accomplishment.

We can't give anyone something we don't have. We must have our own experience of satisfaction before we will ever be able to give satisfaction to another. Giving to yourself in these ways will empower you to give to others in bigger and better ways, creating more and more personal satisfaction and a life full of meaning, purpose, circuitry and continuity.

One thing I have learned is that in order to feel restored and to consistently renew your resources, it is important to connect with like-minded people who also wish to become creators of their own satisfaction, masters of their destiny. I would like to give you this one last tool for your journey. Each week I write a blog, what I call a Shot of Satisfaction, to help put and keep in perspective the tools we need to use in our daily work.

You can sign up to get these at clear2care.com. I invite you to post comments or email me directly with your questions, stories, and so on. You can also follow me on Twitter or join our group page on Facebook, where you can meet and interact with other healthcare heroes on the journey.

In your life and your career in modern medicine, you can have everything you ever dreamed of, and you have to know that it all starts with your wanting more than you already have. If you want more, then you have to leave the place you are in and start the journey to that land of more, the land of plenty: the land of quantum levels of satisfaction.

If you want to feel good and get more out of the life you are living, you have to leave your ordinary day, you ordinary ways and your ordinary thinking and step into your own journey. The first step starts with your desire for more, your desire to feel good (again), to feel good now, to feel good in the future, more and more often. If you believe that there is more to life, that there is a better way, then it's time to take your first step.

Chapter 11

Your Own Quantum Shift

There is an old saying: "Physician, heal thyself." They also say we teach what we need to learn. My own personal healing as a physician started with my desire for more, for something better than what I already had. It seemed to me as if I was working so very hard, but still unable to find what it was I was looking for through my career as an emergency physician. I wanted to feel good about my caring for others. I was so frustrated and numb. I was suffering all the symptoms of burnout. Even outside the hospital, my friendships were eroding; my ability to be intimate with my partner disappeared. I tried and I tried to make things better, but they only got worse. My ultimate healing was born of a tragedy that finally woke me up to the fact that, even though I had devoted my whole life to caring for others, I had not truly cared.

As a result, I became determined to transform tragedy into triumph. I searched for the answer. I knew one existed. I would get better and feel alive again. I would be the phoenix that rose from the ashes, or else. I was out the door and on my way, and I was not coming home until I found what I was looking for, what we are all looking for. What I have shared with you in this book is the journey that followed: my own personal journey through life and medicine, on both sides of the stethoscope.

I discovered that all I ever really wanted from my career, and from life, was to care and be cared for. I realized that my desire to care alone was not enough. I soon understood that I did not know how to care, because I did not really know what care was. As I looked up to the heavens for answers and scoured the literature for clues, I noticed that a key puzzle piece laid in what I was already doing. My first glimpse of the new world I now live in came from recognizing the intense satisfaction I experienced whenever I was fortunate enough to be invited to "step inside the emergency," into extreme situations where all of the distractions from what is important naturally and, more importantly, automatically fall away.

I showed you this with Adam's story. Looking back, I realized it was there that I was able to see how my intense desire to care and save this patient, because of my connection to him and his parents, fueled me to use all of my training and my technical skills to create change for him, for them. Being so completely engaged in the process, giving my all to the situation—including my vulnerabilities—that sort of full engagement could indeed work miracles. Recognizing that this satisfaction was not mine alone— that it involved the whole staff and that it spilled over into the hospital and the community—set the direction my journey would take. I wanted to be a hero all the time!

Heroes all have one thing in common. They are all just people; their special powers lie dormant. They have yet to reach their full human potential—until one day something happens. These ordinary people then go through a process like the intense pressure applied to coal that results in a beautiful diamond. Heroes have to submit to a process very much like that to realize their powers.

Recently, I met a woman at one of the sites I covered who complained from the moment I met her about how she was being treated poorly. She was convinced that her assignment was harder than those of the other nurses. She was angry because she could not get the other nurses to help her. She was totally stuck inside herself, asking me if I could see how she was being mistreated and abused. Listening to her, I realized that she was the "me" from days gone by. She was the "me" who felt that he was working harder than anyone else and he was the only one who cared. She, like the old me, was creating her own negative reality.

Soon things escalated and she was actually verbally sparring with the other nurses. Ultimately the nursing supervisor was summoned to the department. After an hour in the break room with the supervisor, it was not clear if the nurse quit or if she was fired, but she stormed out of the place angry and broken. How I wished she could have read this book. It was like she modeled all the bad behaviors and circuit breakers we have examined here. It was painful to watch her struggle, as I used to struggle all the time. I don't want any of you to struggle so much any longer. You don't have to.

You and I do this work because we want to help, to care, to have our care make a difference. We want to be connected to something larger than ourselves. We do these jobs because we want to be connected to a group of people who want the same. We do these jobs because we want to feel significance in our lives. We do these jobs because we want meaning and purpose. We do these jobs so that at the end of the day we can say we matter and we are doing the important work of helping others.

If this poor nurse could have only applied step one of our framework (to remember why she came to the profession in the first place and reconnect with her desire to care), her situation would have been totally transformed. *She* would have been transformed. I have been totally transformed by the steps I have taken on my own journey, and I have done my best to share these steps to transformation with you. The beauty of applying the R.E.F.L.E.C.T. framework to our daily practice is that if we honestly look into the universal mirror to see who we are, we will, in time, see that our own reflection has changed. We are not the me that we used to be. We will be transformed as individuals and we will transcend our present limited state where we suffer compassion fatigue and burnout. We will once again be happy and satisfied with who we are and what we are doing in our world.

We all get confused on a daily basis between care and cure. We have forgotten to focus on the one thing that we can't touch in our encounters, the energy that will make a difference. Care is not cure. Care is not tangible. True Care is an energetic phenomenon that is simultaneously both a noun and a verb. True Care is generated with our hearts and our minds and delivered one on one, at the bedside. True Care exists only in one place, Einstein's quantum world.

True Care requires us to dismantle the myth that connecting to our patient or their family members in their pain is bad for us and bad for them. Nothing could be further from the truth. Yes it hurts to empathize with someone in an impossible situation. But it is only by stepping freely into their pain that we will be able to take some of that pain away from them and make them feel better by turning on our compassion, our desire for their suffering to end. Until now, most of us have been omitting this step almost completely from the process we use to deliver the goods and services we call healthcare—and when we do this, there is no way we can generate satisfaction on either side of the stethoscope.

I believe that the reason we do this is because we have been taught and warned not to get too close or connect with our patients. We are taught to stay objective and keep a safe clinical distance. We are taught that keeping this distance is good for the patient and good for us. But working in healthcare and leaving out the care is sort of like making widgets for a living. We will never be satisfied with this. Our patients will never be satisfied with this, no matter how incredible the cure we deliver is.

True Care is a simple process. First we get present, then we connect with the person in front of us, make their needs our focus, we make the empathetic connection and we feel their pain as if it were our own, we then turn on and feel our own compassion for them and finally we speak or act from there. It is in the experience of our own compassion that we and our patient begin to feel better and start to get the "more" from life that we are all after.

While this process is quite simple, we need to work to be sure that the care we deliver is clean and simple too, free of attachments or agendas. Turns out that caring for another is relatively easy, until we allow ourselves to judge our patient as undeserving of our care, or not needing our care, or until we see them as demanding our care or feeling entitled to our care, or until we expect a thank you for our care. These are some of the things that can get in the way of our caring. But when we look deeper, we can see how the real obstacles to our caring lie not in our patient or our environment, but within us. We unfortunately, and unconsciously, get in our own way.

In the quantum world of thoughts and emotional energies, the problem is never the situation or person we are encountering. The problem is never out there. The problem is always inside us. The problem is our automatic physiologic reaction: our beast within, our spoiled inner child. We need to use the framework in this book to step out of our own way, to step out of our own automatic physiology and neurochemistry, to clear the judgments and negative thoughts that stop us from really caring for our patients. We need to work with our minds to become clear enough about what we want and what we are doing so that we can generate and deliver True Care.

The truth, as we have come to understand, is that humans are hard-wired to care. The MRI scanner shows us that when we are experiencing compassion, all of the dopamine-rich feel-good centers in our prefrontal cortex actually light up. So it is in our best interest to let go of being right. It is in our best interest to clear our judgments and misconceptions of others. It is in our best interest to reconnect with our pure, simple, uncorrupted desire to care, make a difference, change our world and save our day. It is in our best interest to get clear enough to care.

Nothing in this life comes for free, and anything worth having is worth working for. This work we've chosen is not easy, nor is it supposed to be. We chose to be heroic, and heroes are here to deal with the chaos and craziness that results in human suffering. But we also come armed with the ultimate weapon: our desire to care for those suffering and hurting humans.

This understanding and the tools that you now have will give you what you need to win your daily battles. You won't always win. Some days will be just too darn hard. But those days will become fewer and farther between as you begin to master these tools. By injecting the energies of care into what you're already doing, you will create the home you are looking for in whatever house you find yourself in.

I have spent my whole life searching, reaching and grabbing for something from "out there," something in the physical world that I could get or do that would make everything all right, that would allow me to finally be OK. I believed that being "great" in this world would mean that I was "great." I now see that this is just like a dog trying to catch his tail.

Now, through the process of applying the seven steps of the R.E.F.L.E.C.T framework and writing this book for you, I realize that I need to be reaching and grabbing for something from inside of me, reaching for that spark of greatness that is within, covered by all my garbage, limitations, insecurities and defenses, and tapping into the potential that is already inside me so that the beauty that is my personal essence can shine into the physical world and be reflected back to me in others. This is where real meaning, purpose, happiness and satisfaction live.

I realize that the validation I am looking for can only come from the world of the intangible, from my soul's connection to my highest self, which actually already exists inside me and around me. I was born with a desire to care, a desire to help and make things better. When I make this connection to my desire, nurture this connection and hold onto this connection, I can channel all the benevolent and powerful energies that are contained within my desire to care. These awesome energies can burn away my garbage and limitations so that my essence is finally revealed. This is what allows us to become more than we are today. This is full actualization of the self.

I have come to realize that my job is to love what seems unlovable within myself and in others; to bring compassion, to bring caring, to bring nurturing, to practice human dignity and, above all, to support others on their journeys. I now realize that to be the cause of greatness in this world, all any of us need to do is tap into the greatness that is already inside us, tap into our unique highest selves and allow this essence to shine into the world through caring for others and sharing this great quantum energy with others.

My life in the new world of medicine, in the land of quantum satisfaction, is so very different than the life I used to live. I am so much happier and more content. I am much more resilient. I have more energy and I have more fun. I am finally getting the more from life that I always wanted.

I no longer blame others for my foul mood or my bad day. I have taken total responsibility for my experience at work and in life. I know that if I am frustrated, I just have to go back to the framework and apply it to my situation and my situation will improve. I realize that if I want more or if I want it to be better, it is up to me. That is real freedom. If I don't have what I want, it just means I have to work harder in both Newton's physical world of cure and Einstein's energetic world of care. I finally have the information I need to have it all.

Is it not interesting that a crazy man who was being badgered for sex by imaginary flying purple cows would try to kill me because he felt I did not care, and that this would send me on a relentless search for the key that would release me from my own pain and suffering, my own need and lack, my own living hell? There is an old saying that the cow wants to feed the calf more than the calf wants to suckle. I am grateful to those flying purple cows that were tormenting my patient Joseph that cold dark night, for if it were not for them, I would never have understood and never been able to share what I now know about the healing power found within the milk of human kindness.

As I personally transition from living the comfortable life to living the high life, I realize there is endless goodness, kindness, mercy and compassion available to all of us in the quantum energetic world, and all we have to do to tap into it is reconnect to our desire to care, to make a difference and to save the day. That's the key that unlocks the gate to real and lasting satisfaction on both sides of the stethoscope.

Now that you know what I know, it is time for you to have it all for yourself. When you step onto the floor at work and apply what you have learned in this book to your practice of nursing or medicine, here's what you will find. You will see that you are working with great people. You will naturally be appreciated. You will feel your creativity reemerge. You will once again be doing meaningful work and you will be confident that you make a difference in the world.

You will feel connected. You will feel like you belong to a group, and you will feel significant in that group. You will feel that you are doing your part in the big picture of life. You will be the cause of change in your world and in the lives of those around you. You will find inspiration and value in the same circumstances that seem so bleak to you today. You will look for and find opportunities to care where you once thought care was impossible.

This is your opportunity to have what you have always wanted. With the framework outlined in this book, when you R.E.F.L.E.C.T., you can get that satisfaction and experience your purpose in this world through the work you are already doing. Nothing around you has to change. *You* will change, you will be transformed, and because you have changed, everything and everyone will change around you. You will become the model of the change you want to see in your world. You will always be the cause of your own satisfaction, and you will be able to share that satisfaction with your co-workers, and deliver it to your patients, one human encounter at a time.

Chapter 12

A Final Reflection

I wish I had known long ago how universal the problem of compassion fatigue and burnout in the medical and nursing professions is. But the truth now is that I'm glad I didn't know. I am happy I was ignorant, for had I known that burnout was to be expected, and that I was "normal," I might never have found the determination and resolve to find the solution for all of us. And I firmly believe that there is a solution—that **burnout never needs to happen, and that if it does happen, there is a clear path back to being a joyful and fulfilled human once again**.

The literature about burnout cites all sorts of stressors: unpredictable challenges, sudden death, violence, trauma, overcrowding, high workloads, having to care for multiple critical patients simultaneously, dealing with victims of physical or sexual abuse—including children—and even dealing with emotionally charged families and loved ones. Yes, our work is incredibly stressful, but I am getting excited just hearing the list of stressors. I actually love swimming in that kind of chaos. These are the reasons I chose emergency medicine! They can't be the reasons we burn out.

I've said it throughout the book: humans are hardwired to care. So the problem has got to be in the software. There's a flaw in the programming we've received—a bug that tells us we can't afford to connect and pops up an error message when we get too close. It tells us we must distance ourselves from our patients and their suffering—and that we must teach those who are coming behind us to do the same.

So we do. We teach them, especially when they hit the floor and the bedside, to objectify their patients—to speak about the man in 422 with pancreatic cancer, rather than about Larry, the young father of three, because (knowing that pancreatic cancer is essentially incurable) seeing him as a person would make it difficult to see him and examine him every day. It would make it impossible to face his young wife.

So if we're treating Larry, we begin to shift our focus away from Larry to Larry's lab tests and imaging studies. We become consumed with finding a cure, extending his life, just so that we don't have to feel his pain—to feel *our* pain. This is where we are in medicine today. This is how we have come to confuse the cure with the care. Because we universally are unwilling to step into someone's pain without first doing something about it, we have forgotten about the immense power that is contained within our own capacity for *kara* and our unlimited, unending resource of compassion, which together can generate the milk of human kindness we all crave no matter which side of the stethoscope we find ourselves on.

What I've tried to show you in this book is a different way, a better way. A fix for your software, if you will. In this new scenario, you think of Larry as Larry, not the man in 422. You go to that place of painful energetic connection to Larry's pain and sadness, and you sit in that pain with him. Maybe, in the fullness of your own capacity for *kara*, you cry with him.

But you don't stay there in the pain. Instead, you let your original, deep, pure desire to *care* for Larry come to the fore—and it is in that moment when you turn on your compassion that things get better both for Larry and for you. That's when the pain that you both feel is burned away by the mix of neurochemicals that are flooding your brains, simply because *you* were willing to stay in Larry's pain for one brief moment in time, long enough to generate the (intangible) sweet milk of human kindness.

This is mind over matter. This is how we use our minds to generate and deliver True Care one patient at a time, over and over again over time, and this is what makes *us* matter. This is how we get our mojo back and share our humanity, our life force, our power with others. And this feels incredibly good!

I promised you that I would teach you how to create more and more feel-good moments at work and in life, and that if you practiced the **R.E.F.L.E.C.T**. framework and stayed focused on the process, you might become so accomplished that you'd feel good all the time. Be patient with yourself. Malcolm Gladwell has shown us that becoming a master at anything takes practice—ten thousand hours of it. But know this too: you can create a feel-good moment for yourself the very next time you are at a patient's bedside.

So what I am asking you to do, even though it is in your best interest, will not be natural (at first). As a matter of fact, you will naturally be afraid to try it. What if, God forbid, you break down and start crying in a patient's room? What if you naturally reach out and wrap your arm around someone who is sobbing hysterically at the news you have just delivered?

What I am asking you to do goes against everything you have ever been taught. Studies show uniformly that doctors take about 10 years to embrace a new drug or technology, so I am praying that using this six-phase protocol for True Care makes you feel so incredibly better that it sparks a desire for you to do it again. I am betting that like me, you will become addicted to that powerful chicken soup of neurotransmitters that bathes your prefrontal cortex in feel-good dopamine each time you turn on and feel the full power of your own compassion, that you will want more, and more . . . and even more.

Initially, pick the patients that are easy to connect with. The woman with confusion and a UTI who reminds you of your Aunt Evelyn or the man with CHF and Gout who reminds you of your Uncle Paul. Pick the cantankerous old goat who reminds you of your grandpa, who refuses to stay in the hospital because he is afraid of losing control, who would rather be at home with the only thing left in his life that shows him any love, his chocolate lab, Rex. Pick the student from the local college with the broken ankle, who reminds you of your nephew, who is at the college on a football scholarship. Pick the young mother who reminds you of your sister, whose child just had a febrile seizure for the first time. Pick the young man who has metastatic testicular cancer on his CXR, who reminds you of me.

If you apply the six stage protocol for generating and delivering True Care with these patients, you can't even imagine how good you will feel, and how satisfying the patient experience is for them, even if there was no valet parking at the ambulatory entrance to your department. By starting with these folks, you will naturally start to get good at and want to apply all the information you have learned through reading this book.

You will show yourself that it really does not add any time to the encounter, and it may in fact shorten the time you spend at the bedside with a particular patient, especially if they are unhappy or unsatisfied and you have to go back in the room and do your best service-excellence dance or speak your best service-recovery rap.

Avoid finding an excuse not to do it. This is not just another level of performance layered onto what you already do. **This is the real essence of who you are and who you really want to be**. This, in fact, is the only thing that can really set you free to be the best physician or nurse, or medic, or tech, or secretary, or husband, wife, lover, sister, brother uncle, or friend, that you can possibly be. True Care can and will change you—forever.

Finally, there will be barriers and roadblocks standing in your way, making you not want to care: The patient who is a jerk. The Malingerer. The Drug Seeker. The Entitled. There are all sorts of patients who will make it difficult for you to care. Save the application of the protocol for these patients until you have a good feel how to use it in other, less challenging situations. But your end game is to always find a way to care. Think of it this way: the harder you have to play the game, the sweeter the victory in the end.

If you're reading this before your shift, that feel-good moment may not even be very many moments away. It's going to be a moment like you have not experienced in years. A moment that will energize you and ignite your desire to create more of the same for yourself, for your patients and for everyone you work with. You have everything you need to do that right now! Here it the first thing to do once you finish this, pick one, just one! Nothing will happen unless you start with one. Remember this: "**The only way out is in.**"

The only way out of your own PTSD, your compassion fatigue, your own burnout, your own depression and hopelessness, you own irritation, anger or dysfunction, is to step into the pain and suffering of another. It's the only way—but you, you are special, you were born with a pure and simple desire to care and make things better, and you were born hardwired to care, so you have everything you need to jump into the fire without getting burned. **Your protection is your compassion**. Turn it on, let it flow, and this mindful act of yours will change everything in (y)our world.

Now go, and share the joy. Take one last look in the mirror before you hit the floor and the patient's bedside and realize **that it is your own R.E.F.L.E.C.T.-ion that has the power to change lives, especially your own**. It's time to remove the warning label. Not only is it now **safe to care**, but it is in (y)our own best interest to care again!

Namaste—

Dr. Frank Gabrin